The Easy Renal Diet Cookbook

100+ Delicious Renal Diet Meals To Improve Kidney Function

JEAN SIMMONS

Copyright © 2019 Jean Simmons

All rights reserved. No part of this publication may be reproduced, distributed, or transmitted in any form or by any means, including photocopying, recording, or other electronic or mechanical methods, without the prior written permission of the publisher, except in the case of brief quotations embodied in critical reviews and certain other noncommercial uses permitted by copyright law.

Limit of Liability/Disclaimer of Warranty: While the publisher and author have used their best efforts in preparing this book, they make no representations or warranties with respect to the accuracy or completeness of the contents of this book and specifically disclaim any implied warranties of merchantability or fitness for a particular purpose. No warranty may be created or extended by sales representatives or written sales materials. The advice and strategies contained herein may not be suitable for your situation. You should consult with a professional where appropriate. Neither the publisher nor author shall be liable for any loss of profit or any other commercial damages, including but not limited to special, incidental, consequential, or other damages

ISBN: 9781092846134

TABLE OF CONTENTS

Also By Jean Simmons 8
INTRODUCTION 1
   The Renal Diet 3
      Controlling Protein 3
      Controlling Potassium 4
      Controlling Phosphorus 6
      Controlling Sodium 7
      Controlling Fluids 9
BREAKFAST 11
   Breakfast Recipes 12
      Simple Breakfast Crostini 12
      Cinnamon French Toast 14
      Hot Tofu Scramble 16
      Pepper-Rich Quiche 18
      Blueberry Pancakes 19
      Mac And Cheese 21
      Green Onion Omelet 22
      Stuffed Breakfast Biscuits 23
      Eggs And Chorizo Burritos 24
      Scrambled Eggs 25
      Laksa Baguette 26
      Mexican Brunch Eggs 27
      Green Chili & Cheese Omelet 29
      Blueberry Muffins 31

    Apple Muffins 33

    Simple Baked Pancakes 34

    Fruit And Oat Pancakes 36

    TexMex Egg & Tortilla 37

    Buttermilk Pancakes 38

    Baked Apple Oatmeal 39

    Multigrain Breakfast Cereal 41

    Bran Muffins 42

LUNCH 45

  Sandwiches & Burgers 46

    Parsley Burger 46

    Couscous Patties 47

    Chicken Burgers 49

    Chili Grilled Cheese Sandwich 51

    Herb Beef Patties 53

    Baked Chicken Broccoli Pizza 54

  Chicken Dishes 57

    Chicken Tikka 57

    Chicken Schnitzel & Rice Cutlets 58

    Spicy Curried Chicken 60

    Chicken Noodle Pancakes 62

  Seafood Dishes 64

    Herb Topped Fish 64

    Baked lemon & Paprika Halibut 66

    White Thatched Cod 67

    Tuna Delight 69

- Pan Fried Stuffed Fish 70
- Salmon And Chive Pate 72
- Smoky Salmon Dip 73

Salad Dishes 75
- Chicken & Rice Salad 75
- Summer Pasta Salad 76
- Cranberry Frozen Salad 78
- Salmon Salad 79
- Macaroni Salad 80
- Shrimp Macaroni Salad 82
- Orzo Salad 83

Vegetable Dishes 84
- Super Lunch Bowl 84
- Crispy Fried Okra 86
- Vegetable Cutlets 87
- Mashed Gingered Carrots 89
- Parmesan & Herb Sautéed Zucchini 90
- Mediterranean Green Beans 92
- Garlic Potato Mash 93
- Summer Vegetable Sauté 94
- Quick Chickpea Curry 95

Couscous 97
- Moroccan Couscous 97
- Mint Couscous 98
- Lemon & Coriander Couscous 99

DINNER 101

- Chicken Dishes 102
  - Chicken With Dill & Honey Sauce 102
  - Moroccan Honey Chicken 104
  - Chicken Stew 106
  - Chicken Mole 107
  - Chicken With Mustard Sauce 109
  - Chicken Sweetcorn Stir Fry 111
  - Chicken And Gnocchi Dumplings 112
  - Chicken With Orange And Ginger 114
  - Chicken Veronique 116
  - Cranberry Spareribs 118
  - Egg Fried Rice 120
  - Pork Stir-Fry With Noodles 122
  - Cranberry Pork Roast 123
  - Pork Chops 125
  - Pork Chops With Herb Crust 126
  - Pork With Pear Chutney 127
- Beef Main Dishes 129
  - Beef & Mushroom Casserole 129
  - Onion- Packed Steak 131
  - Texas Hash 133
  - Spicy Beef Stir-Fry 134
  - Beef And Barley Stew 136
  - Savory Mince 137
  - BBQ Baby Back Ribs 139
  - Low Sodium Pizza 141

    Beef Casserole 143

    Chili Rice With Beef 144

    Peppercorn Steak 146

  Seafood Main Dishes 147

    Salmon Mornay 147

    Tuna & Lemon Pasta 149

    Cod Fillet With Lemon Sauce 151

    Spicy Pesto Catfish 152

SNACKS & DESSERTS 155

  Snacks 156

    Spicy Apple Juice 156

    Fresh Fruit Compote 157

    Garlic Oyster Crackers 158

  Desserts 160

    Baked Custard 160

    Chinese Almond Cookies 162

    Low Sodium Pound Cake 164

    Cinnamon Crisps 165

    Chocolate Strawberries 166

    Vanilla Ice Cream 167

    Maple Crisp Bars 169

    Cinnamon Rice Pudding 171

    Strawberry Ice Cream 173

Also By Jean Simmons

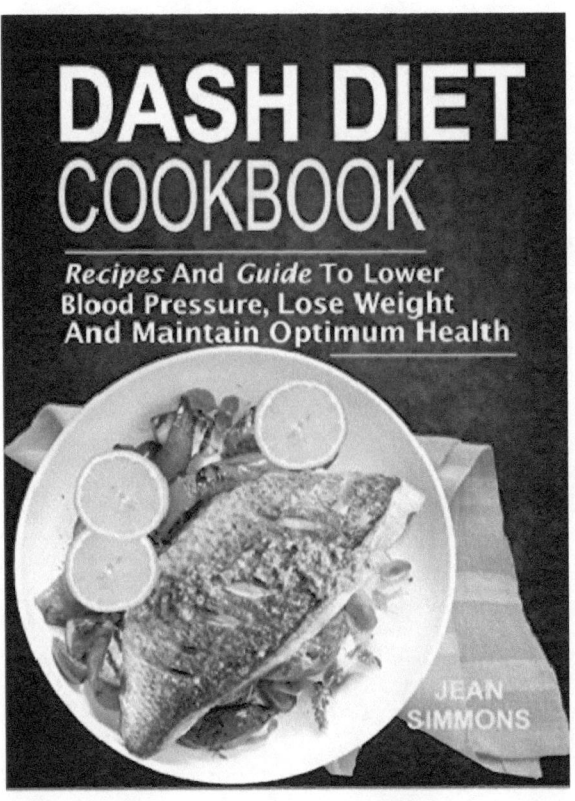

Dash Diet Cookbook: Recipes And Guide To Lower Blood Pressure, Lose Weight And Maintain Optimum Health

INTRODUCTION

Renal disease, chronic kidney disease, renal failure or kidney failure describes a loss of kidney function. When this happens, the kidneys cannot carry out their main function of filtering out wastes and fluids from the blood. People with failing kidneys must follow a renal diet to significantly lower the amount of wastes in their blood. This wastes comes from the food we eat. Renal diet also helps their kidneys to function better and prevents a complete and permanent damage of their kidneys. A renal diet is a diet that is designed to control the intake of fluids, sodium, phosphorus, potassium and protein, depending on individual conditions.

People with kidney disease must ensure that they control the level of chemicals and fluids that enter into their body. Since their kidneys are failing, they cannot process excess liquid. Even with the help of dialysis (artificial kidney treatments), it is impossible to remove all the waste and fluids that build up in the body. This is why they must follow a renal diet to limit the buildup of waste products in their body. The renal diet is restrictive. The amount of essential nutrients, such as protein, sodium, potassium, phosphorus and fluids that enter the body must be controlled. These are the nutrients that can affect the kidneys.

No potassium for instance, means no bananas, no yams, few tomatoes, few nuts, and a negligible amount of coconut milk. The versatile dietary staple, potatoes, must be boiled, drained and re-cooked to remove or significantly lower its high potassium content. No sodium means no salt. Additionally, if sufferers are diabetic as well, they must also limit carbs, sugar and fruits in their diet and restrict fat as well. Fluids must also be limited. They must reduce the liquid in their foods and drinks. Some resort to sucking ice cubes to alleviate thirst. This makes the renal diet not only restrictive, but inconvenient. This is because, many sufferers often sacrifice taste and pleasure for necessity.

The truth is that isn't that difficult to find delicious meals that you and your family will love. It is simply a case of modifying recipes to produce tasty and flavorful meals. This book makes the balance between enjoying your meals and making the right adjustments necessary for your health. The recipes are delicious and contain nutritional facts that discloses the quantities of salt, potassium and phosphate in a serving. The wide range of recipes are quick and easy to make with everyday ingredients, which are affordable as well. They all contain suitable serving sizes, with suitable amount of salt, phosphate, potassium and fluid. Furthermore, the book provides hints, tips and ideas to add creativity to your meals.

However, not everyone will have the same restrictions. Some may need to limit calcium. Some patients need only to reduce fluids, before starting dialysis. Others need to eat high-quality protein foods once dialysis is started. Every person's body is different and so people have individual diet requirements. If you have kidney disease, your diet may be different from another person.

It is extremely important that you work with your renal dietician to guide you in the best meal plan that is suitable for you. Factors such as your weight, age, dialysis treatment, as well as medical conditions, such as diabetes, high blood pressure and heart disease will be thoroughly considered. Your dietician will ensure that your diet is tailored to address your specific need. It is only by following the right diet that you can get your kidneys to work for as long as possible.

The Renal Diet

Diet is an integral part of treating kidney disease. Your meal must contain a good balance of calories from different food sources to keep your body healthy.

Controlling Protein
Protein helps to build muscles and repair tissues. It is important to eat the right amount of protein and the right kind as well. Why? So your kidneys will be protected. Our kidneys help to remove waste from protein that the body uses. The right amount of protein in your body will guard against infections and prevent wastes from accumulating in your blood. Eating large portions of protein may overwork the kidneys. Therefore, it is best to eat small portion sizes of protein foods (e.g. ½ cup of yoghurt or milk per serving or 2- 3 ounces of protein per serving). But if on dialysis, you'll need more.

There are 2 kinds of protein sources. The best protein sources are from animal products. They include meats, fish, eggs, poultry and dairy products. Others come from vegetables and grains such as beans, legumes and tofu. To enjoy a balanced diet, both kinds of proteins should be included in daily meals. Nevertheless, check with your dietician on the right protein combinations that is suitable for you.

Controlling Potassium

Potassium is a mineral found in foods. It regulates nerves and helps the muscles to work right. It is also important for heart function. The kidneys help to maintain the right amount of potassium in the body, by removing excess potassium through urination. But when the kidneys break down, it can no longer remove potassium and the potassium builds up in the blood. This is dangerous. If the potassium level gets too high, it may lead to irregular heartbeats or even a heart attack. A normal blood potassium level is 3.5-5.0. If is too low, supplements can help raise it. If too high, staying away from high potassium foods will greatly help. The average healthy individual requires about 3500 to 4500 milligrams of potassium per day. However, only about 2000 milligrams per day is required for people with kidney disease.

All foods contain potassium; but some foods contain higher amounts than others. High potassium foods include: bananas, avocadoes, peas and dried beans. Tomatoes, tomato juice, tomato purees, oranges, winter squash and cantaloupe. Dried fruits, milk, chocolates, nuts, prunes and potatoes. Low potassium foods include: Alfalfa sprouts, cabbage, cauliflower, mixed vegetables, eggplant, zucchini squash, corn and broccoli. Rice, noodles, pasta, bread and berries, pineapples, apples, grapes and pears. Double-boiling or soaking vegetables reduces the amount of potassium in them.

It is possible to include some high potassium foods in your diet. But as earlier mentioned, you have to leach them before using. Leaching helps to pull out of some of the potassium contained in vegetables; but it cannot pull out all. You still have to eat a moderate amount of leached high-potassium vegetables. Consult your renal dietitian on the amount of leached high potassium vegetables that are safe to include in your diet.

Additionally, the portion serving of the food you eat is important. Eating a large amount of low potassium food could end up becoming a high-potassium one. This is why it is important to consult your renal dietician who will help you to plan your diet to ensure you get the appropriate amount of potassium needed in a day. Factors such as how well your kidneys are functioning and certain medications you might be taking will also have to be put into consideration.

Leaching Potatoes, Sweet Potatoes, Beets, Carrots and Winter Squash:

1. Peel the vegetables and place in cold water to prevent darkening.

2. Slice them about 1/8 thick and rinse in warm water.

3. Soak in lots of warm water for at least 2 hours. The water should be 10 times more than the quantity of vegetables.

4. Rinse again under warm water and then cook with lots of water. This should be 5 times more than the amount of vegetables being cooked.

Controlling Phosphorus

Phosphorus is a mineral present in the bones that helps to form strong bones and teeth. It works with calcium to achieve this function. Phosphorus also helps to maintain an acid/base balance in the body. Healthy kidneys remove excess phosphorus present in the blood. But in kidneys that are aren't working well, phosphorus starts to build up in the blood. To balance these minerals, the body pulls calcium out of your bones into the blood, weakening the bones. Once the phosphorus and calcium bind together in the blood, they can deposits in the blood vessels, skin, lungs, joints and eyes. This is dangerous and may damage the heart and other vital organs; cause bone pain and aches; poor blood circulation; and skin ulcers.

Phosphorus is found in most foods. However, large amounts of it are present in: dairy products (cheese, milk, pudding, ice cream and yogurt); Protein (oysters, sardines, chicken & beef liver, fish roe); beverages (colas, cocoa, ale, beer); Whole grains, (especially bran); Nuts, seeds, lentils and beans. Avoid foods with phosphorus addictive as well. Limiting these high phosphorus foods will help to keep your phosphorus levels in check. A normal phosphorus level is 2.5 to 4.5 mg/dL. If you have kidney disease, your diet is usually limited to a daily consumption of 1000 mg of phosphorus.

Have just 1 serving of 7 ounces when eating meats and fish. Do not exceed 1 serving of 4 ounces when taking milk and other dairy products. Use non-dairy creamers instead of milk to lower the amount of phosphorus in your diet.

There are medications for phosphorus control called a phosphate binder. They help to control the amount of phosphorus absorbed by your body. They come in form of pills, powders, chewable tablets, and liquids. Some contain calcium as well. Your doctor or dietitian will prescribe the phosphate binder that is best for you, which will be taken your meal.

Controlling Sodium

Sodium is a mineral that helps to regulate the water content in your body. It is found naturally in foods, but often high in table salts. Failing kidneys cause extra sodium and fluids to build up in the body. This may lead to high blood pressure, puffiness, fluids in the hearts and lungs, shortness of breath and swollen ankles. Most of the sodium that we eat comes from cured and processed foods. Food manufacturers often add sodium in high amounts to certain foods. A healthy diet should include 1500 to 2000mg of sodium in a day. Therefore, limit your amount of salt and salt seasonings; salty foods; cured foods; luncheon meats and processed foods.

To limit your sodium intake:

Avoid:

- Table salt and any "salt" seasonings.
- Salt substitutes because they contain high amounts of potassium.
- Salty meats or smoked meats (hot dogs, ham, sausage, bacon, canned meats, or bologna).
- Salty snacks (salted crackers, pretzels and chips).
- Canned soups, mustard, ketchup, meat tenderizers instant noodles and frozen dinners, bottled sauces, olives, pickles, and MSG.
- Packaged foods and restaurant foods.
- Smoked meats and smoked or processed cheeses.

Instead:

- Cook with herbs, spices, lemon juice or vinegar instead of salt.
- Eat foods closest to their natural, unprocessed state.

- Read food labels and buy foods low in sodium.
- When eating out, order for meat or fish without salt.
- Prepare foods from scratch, to help control the amount of sodium used.

Checking package Labels For Sodium

Go through the package label. Read the sodium information on it. Sodium is too high if salt is listed in the first five ingredients. Additionally, check the serving size and weigh it with your recommended total daily allowance. Food labels have milligrams (mg) of sodium listed. 1000 mg is equal to 1g. Therefore, If your diet allows you to have 2 grams of sodium per day. Then you mustn't exceed 2000 milligrams. If a sodium level per serving is 500mg or more, avoid the food item as the sodium content is too high. Check the labels of similar food products and pick the one that has the lowest sodium level for the same serving size.

When reading labels, you must understand the terms generally used. They include:

Sodium Free: This means only an insignificant amount per serving.

Reduced Sodium: This means the level of sodium in the foods is reduced by 25%.

Low Sodium: This means 140 mg or less per serving.

Very Low Sodium: Indicates 35 mg or less per serving.

Light in Sodium – The means the sodium in the foods is reduced by at least 50%.

Controlling Fluids

Fluid is important for all body functions. Our body needs the right amount of water (about 8 glasses) to maintain fluid balance. But restrictions may be necessary for people with kidney failure, especially those at the last stages of chronic kidneys. This is because the kidneys whose job is to help maintain fluid balance isn't working well. Excess fluid in the body can lead to breathlessness, (caused by fluid on your lungs) high blood pressure, headaches, and puffy eyes. People on dialysis do not pass out urine as often as they should.

Fluid restrictions vary for patients. If you have kidney disease, your fluid intake should be monitored with the help of your nurse. Your weight determines the amount of fluid that you require. Your doctor uses your weight to assess the amount of fluid that you are losing. If monitoring fluid intake, record them in a fluid balance chart.

Tips for managing your thirst & restricting fluids:

- Stay cool!
- Avoid salt- do not add salt to foods, eat less salty foods and avoid processed foods.
- Limit consumption of certain foods that have high water content. Examples include watermelon, gravy, soup, and ice cream.
- Drink cold liquids instead of hot beverages.
- Take small sips and not big gulps. Use small cups for your beverages.
- Take your medicines with your meal; swallow pills with applesauce, and not water.
- Try sucking small ice cubes. Freeze approved fruit juices in ice trays for a special treat.
- If your mouth feels dry, try taking certain sweets like mints, hard candy or chewing gum, instead of water.

- If you have diabetes, maintaining a blood glucose levels will keep your thirst in check. High blood glucose levels increases thirst.

Other helpful hints:

- Do not drink the liquid from canned fruits and vegetables. Steer clear of juices from cooked meats as well.
- Always check the ingredients in the recipe - check the potassium, phosphate, salt and fluid level of each ingredient in a recipe.
- Par-boil vegetables before cooking to reduce the potassium content. Use fresh products instead of tinned.
- Instead of using liquid stock or stock cubes, use homemade stock made from vegetables and meat bones with low potassium content.

BREAKFAST

Breakfast is essential for everyone, particularly for people with kidney failure or Chronic Kidney Disease (CKD). Breakfast provide the energy that is needed to face the day. It improves concentration, reduces stress and generally makes you feel better.

Do not make a habit of skipping it. For doing so may result in adverse health effects such as diabetes and high cholesterol, which can increase the risk of kidney failure after a period of time. Even in sleep, your body is at work; therefore, when you wake up, take breakfast within 2 hours to replenish the nourishment that your body lost. Eating breakfast also reduces hunger pangs that will inevitably occur in the course of the day, resulting in overeating at lunch or dinner.

Ideal breakfast for kidney failure includes foods high in fiber and protein such as natural cereals, whole grain cereals, and high fiber cereals from unrefined carbohydrates are best. Oats, boiled egg with whole grain toast. Below is an interesting collection of renal breakfast recipes that will help your kidneys to function better, while providing you with the satisfaction and nourishment that you need.

Breakfast Recipes

Simple Breakfast Crostini
A great breakfast idea that can also work with stale bread or almost any type of bread, apart from pre-sliced. Also, all the vegetables must be pre-cooked.

Prep Time: 10 minutes

Cook Time: 10 minutes

Serves: 4

Ingredients

1 wholemeal baguette, cut into 16 slices of ½ inch thickness

8 cherry tomatoes, sliced

1 red pepper, sliced thinly

4 mushrooms, sliced

1/3 cup of cooked spinach, squeezed of water

1 slice of lean ham, strips

2 spring onions, sliced thinly

2 eggs, scrambled

¾ cup of reduced-fat cheddar, grated finely

Directions

1. Prepare all the toppings ingredients.

2. Toast a side of the bread slices on a grill pan. Remove and flip bread slices to grill the other side.

3. Arrange the toppings on the bread; make a couple of each type of crostini and sprinkle with grated cheddar.

4. Grill until almost brown.

Nutritional Facts Per Serving: 1portion of fruit & veggies

Calories: 294

Potassium: 279mg

Sodium: 268mg

Protein: 15.7g

Carbohydrates: 35.3g

Fat: 11g

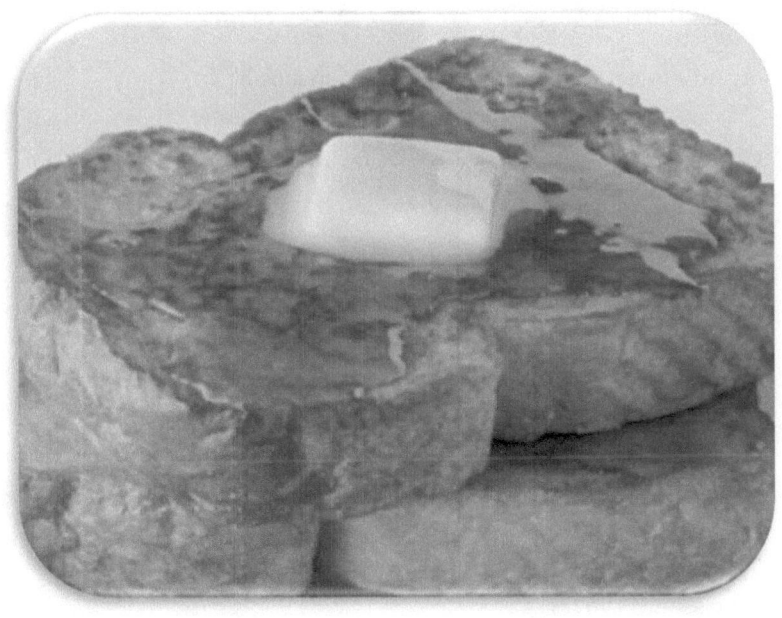

Cinnamon French toast with cinnamon syrup

Cinnamon French Toast

Prep Time: 5 minutes

Cook Time: 10 minutes

Serves: 3

Ingredients

2 eggs, slightly beaten

6 slices raisin bread

3/4 cup of light non- dairy creamer, non- fortified

Cooking spray

Cinnamon

Directions

1. Add together the creamer and eggs in a dish.

2. Coat both sides of bread slices in the egg mixture by dipping and turning.

3. Spray pan with non-stick spray and brown one side of the bread with cinnamon.

4. Turn the other side and brown, adding more cook spray, if necessary, so it doesn't stick.

5. Enjoy with 1/2 cup of applesauce.

Nutritional Facts Per Serving: 2 slices

Calories: 229

Potassium: 196 mg

Phosphorus: 91 mg

Sodium: 337 mg

Calcium: 76mg

Protein: 7 g

Calcium: 66 mg

Carbohydrates: 30 g

Fat: 8 g

Cholesterol: 101mg

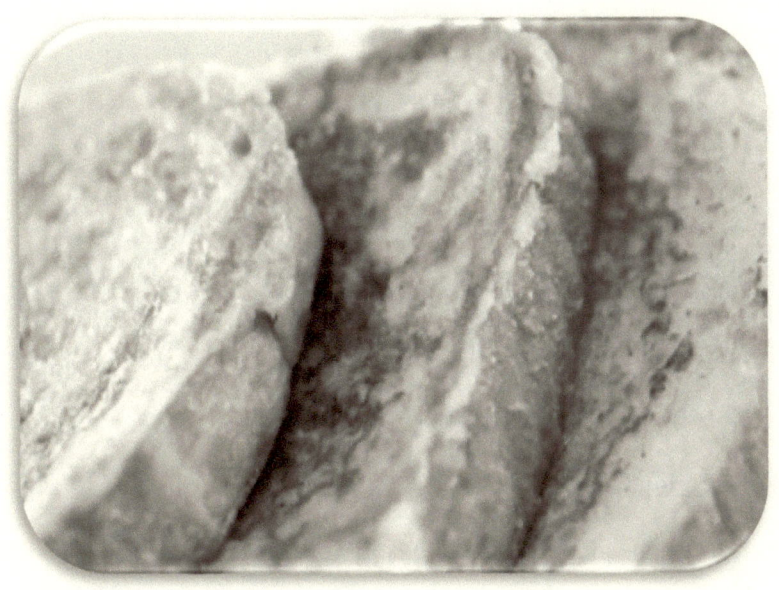

Cinnamon French toast

Hot Tofu Scramble

A vegan breakfast option that's packed with spices and vegetables. For your Tofu, go through the nutritional label and buy the one that's less than 10% calcium.

Prep Time: 10 minutes

Cook Time: 10 minutes

Serves: 2

Ingredients

1 teaspoon olive oil

¼ cup green bell pepper, chopped

¼ cup red bell pepper, chopped

1 cup firm tofu

¼ teaspoon garlic powder

1 teaspoon onion powder

1 clove garlic, minced

⅛ teaspoon of turmeric

Directions

1. In a non- stick skillet, add the olive oil, the bell peppers and garlic and sauté.

2. Rinse the tofu and crumble it into the skillet and then add the rest of the ingredients.

3. Let it cook, with frequent stir, on low heat for about 20 minutes, until the tofu becomes slightly golden brown in color. Water will evaporate as well.

4. Enjoy warm!

Nutritional Facts Per Serving: 1 serving = ½ cup

Calories: 213

Potassium: 467 mg

Phosphorus: 242 mg

Sodium: 24mg

Protein: 15.7g

Carbohydrates: 10g

Fat: 13g

Calcium: 274 mg

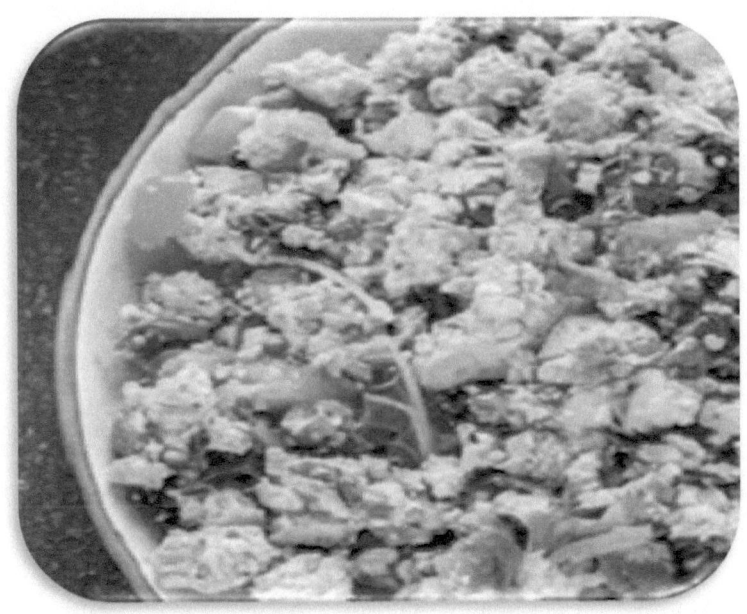

Pepper-Rich Quiche

Prep Time: 10 minutes

Cook Time: 60 minutes

Serves: 8

Ingredients

1 tablespoon margarine

1 green pepper, sliced

1 sweet red pepper, sliced

1 sweet yellow pepper, sliced

4 eggs

1/2 cup liquid non-dairy creamer

1/8 teaspoon of cayenne pepper

1/2 teaspoon basil

1 9-inch pie shell, unbaked

1/2 cup water

Directions:

1. Melt the margarine in a large skillet, place in the pepper strips and sauté until tender.

2. In a bowl, add together the eggs, creamer, basil, cayenne and water.

3. Use a spoon to put the peppers into the unbaked pie shell.

4. Place in the oven to bake at 375°F for 50- 60 minutes.

5. Let it rest for 10 minutes before serving.

Nutritional Facts Per Serving: 1/8 Quiche Per Serving

Calories: 201

Potassium: 163 mg; Phosphorus: 50 mg; Sodium: 222mg

Protein: 5g; Carbohydrates: 14g; Fat: 14g

Blueberry Pancakes

Prep Time: 10minutes

Cook Time: 20minutes

Serves: 12

Ingredients

1½ cups all-purpose flour, sifted

2 teaspoons of baking powder

3 tablespoons of sugar

1 cup buttermilk

2 eggs, slightly beaten

1 cup frozen blueberries, rinsed

2 tablespoons of unsalted margarine, melted

Directions

1. In a mixing bowl, sift together the flour and the baking powder, together with the sugar.

2. Make a deep hole in the center and place in the rest of the ingredients. Stir to smoothen.

3. Place a large pan on heat and then grease lightly. Scoop ½ cup of batter into the pan, cook and flip until cooked to desired doneness.

Nutritional Facts Per Serving: 2 pancakes per serving

Calories: 223

Potassium: 100mg

Phosphorus: 242mg

Sodium: 196mg

Protein: 7g

Carbohydrates: 35g

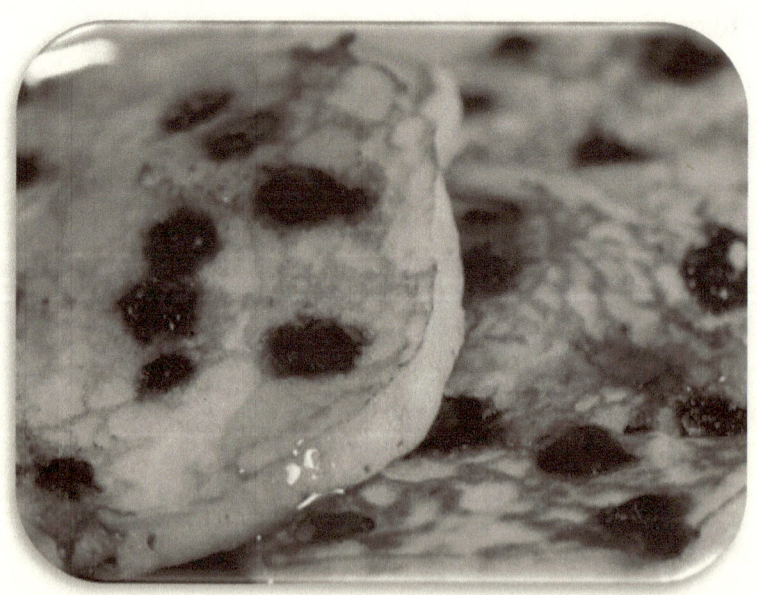

Mac And Cheese

Enjoy this low sodium macaroni and cheese for breakfast.

Prep Time: 5minutes

Cook Time: 15minutes

Serves: 4

Ingredients

1/4 teaspoon of mustard, dried

1 teaspoon of unsalted margarine

1/2 cup of grated cheddar cheese

2 cups of noodles of choice

2-3 cups hot water

Directions

1. Cook the noodles in the hot water for about 5 minutes or until softened.

2. Drain the noodles and top immediately with the grated cheese, butter and mustard. Stir to mix well.

3. Place in the oven and bake for about 10 minutes at a temperature of 350°F until the top is slightly golden brown.

Nutritional Facts Per Serving:

Calories: 163

Potassium: 39 mg; Phosphorus: 138 mg; Sodium: 114 mg

Protein: 6g; Carbohydrates: 20 g

Green Onion Omelet

Prep Time: 2 minutes

Cook Time: 5minutes

Serves: 1

Ingredients

2 eggs, beaten slightly

3 tablespoons of milk, 2%

2 tablespoons of green onions, chopped

Dash of pepper

2 teaspoons butter or margarine

Directions

1. Add the pepper and milk to the slightly beaten eggs in a bowl.

2. Melt the butter in a skillet and then add the egg mixture. Let it cook for a few minutes.

3. Fold one half of the egg, over the other.

Nutritional Facts Per Serving:

Calories: 322

Potassium: 303 mg

Phosphorus: 170 mg

Sodium: 209 mg; Calcium: 322 mg

Protein: 20g; Carbohydrates: 4g,

Fat: 24 g, Cholesterol: 640mg

Stuffed Breakfast Biscuits

Prep Time: 5minutes

Cook Time: 10minutes

Serves: 1

Ingredients

2 cups flour

1 tablespoon honey

1 tablespoon lemon juice

1/2 teaspoon baking soda

8 tablespoons or1 stick softened butter

3/4 cup milk

For the filling:

4 eggs, scrambled, (about 1 cup cooked)

¾ cup or 8-oz pack crisp, uncured bacon, coarsely chopped

1 cup cheddar cheese

¼ cup scallions, thinly sliced

Directions

1. Preheat your oven to 425°F.

2. Add together all the dry ingredients in large bowl.

3. Cut the butter in with a pastry cutter until smaller. Create a well in center, add the milk and knead. Gently fold in the filling and then press dough into a ball.

4. Bake for 10 minutes or until it is golden brown.

Nutritional Facts Per Serving: Calories: 304

Potassium: 122mg; Phosphorus: 147mg; Sodium: 235mg

Protein: 9g; Calcium: 322mg; Carbohydrates: 19g

Fat: 2g; Cholesterol: 106mg

Eggs And Chorizo Burritos

A delicious and satisfying breakfast on the go!

Prep Time: 5minutes

Cook Time: 10minutes

Serves: 3

Ingredients

3 ounces of Mexican sausage (chorizo)

3 flour tortillas

3 eggs, beaten

Directions

1. Place the chorizo in a skillet and sauté until dark in color.

2. Add the beaten eggs, stir and cook until done.

3. Next, warm the tortillas and fill up with the fried mixture. Fold up the bottom edge and roll up so it does not fall out.

Nutritional Facts Per Serving: Calories: 320

Potassium: 214 mg; Phosphorus: 170 mg; Sodium: 659 mg

Protein: 16 g; Calcium: 66 mg; Carbohydrates: 18 g; Fat: 20 g

Scrambled Eggs

Prep Time: 5 minutes

Cook Time: 5 minutes

Serves: 1

Ingredients

2 large eggs, beaten

1 teaspoon dried dill weed

1/8 teaspoon black pepper

1 tablespoon of crumbled goat cheese

Directions

1. Add the beaten eggs, dill weed and black pepper in a nonstick skillet and cook over medium heat.

2. Once the eggs are scrambled, top with the crumbled goat cheese.

3. Serve immediately!

Nutritional Facts Per Serving: 2 eggs

Calories: 194

Potassium: 192 mg; Phosphorus: 250 mg; Sodium: 213 mg

Protein: 16 g; Calcium: 214 mg; Carbohydrates: 1 g; Fat: 14g

Laksa Baguette

Prep Time: 5 minutes

Cook Time: 5 minutes

Serves: 1

Ingredients

1 baguette slice, 1 inch thick

1/4 onion, chopped

1 egg, beaten

1/4 can tuna

1 pinch salt

1 dash turmeric powder

1/2 teaspoon chili paste

3 laksa leaves, chopped finely

Directions

1. Combine the tuna and the beaten egg together in a bowl.

2. Add the onions, chili and turmeric powder in a pan and fry until translucent.

3. Add in the egg mixture, fry and stir.

4. Sprinkle the laksa leaves over the hot egg.

5. Enjoy with a slice of baguette.

Nutritional Facts Per Serving: 2 eggs

Calories: 259

Sodium: 358 mg; Protein: 21 g; Carbohydrates: 16 g

Fat: 13g; Cholesterol: 164mg

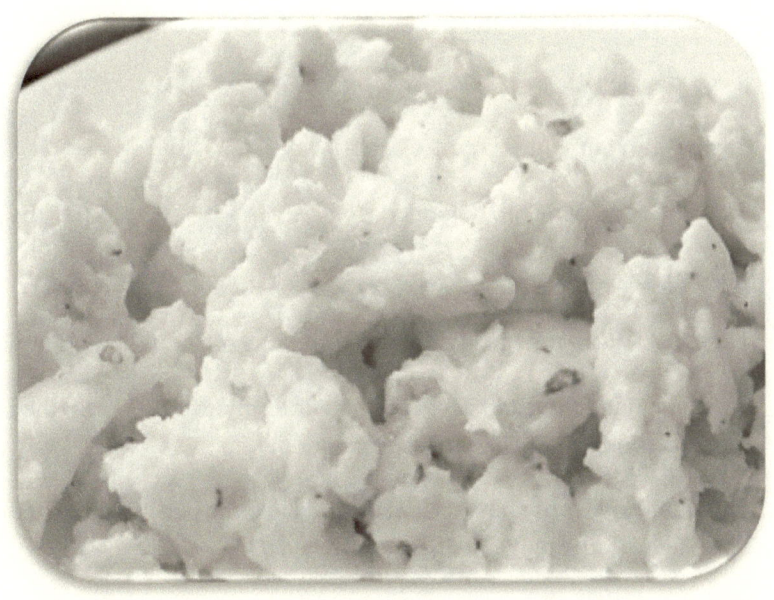

Scrambled eggs

Mexican Brunch Eggs

Prep Time: 5 minutes

Cook Time: 10minutes

Serves: 8

Ingredients

1/2 cup onion, chopped

2 tablespoons margarine

2 cloves garlic, crushed

1 1/2 teaspoons ground cumin

1 1/2 cups frozen corn, thawed

1/8 teaspoon cayenne pepper

8 eggs, beaten

2 cups corn chips, unsalted

2 tablespoons pimiento, chopped

Directions:

1. Melt the margarine in a skillet and sauté the garlic and onion until tender.

2. Add cumin, corn, and cayenne and stir to mix well. Pour in the beaten egg and cook, with occasional stirring, until set.

3. Arrange the corn chips on a plate and ladle the egg mixture over it. Sprinkle with the pimiento. Serve and enjoy!

Nutritional Facts Per Serving: 1/2 cup per serving

Calories: 214

Potassium: 240 mg

Phosphorus: 91 mg

Sodium: 147 mg

Protein: 9 g

Calcium: 214 mg

Carbohydrates: 13 g

Fat: 14g

Green Chili & Cheese Omelet

Prep Time: 5 minutes

Cook Time: 5 minutes

Serves: 4

Ingredients

4 eggs

1 tablespoon of butter or margarine

4 tablespoons of water

4 oz. Monterrey jack cheese, cut in strips

1 4-oz can of green chilies, peeled, drained & rinsed

For the sauce:

1 tablespoon of butter

1/4 cup of canned, no sodium added tomatoes, drained and chopped

Directions

1. Place the butter in a skillet and melt over medium heat.

2. In a bowl, beat the eggs and add the water, whisking until foamy.

3. Add the egg mixture to the pan, set heat to low and use a spatula to run around the edges. Lift up so that the uncooked egg mixture can flow under.

4. Now wrap the chilies around the strip of cheese and place on one half of the omelet. Use spatula to loosen the edges and fold over.

5. Make the sauce by melting the butter in a pan, adding the chopped onion and tomatoes, simmering for about 5 minutes.

6. Pour sauce over the omelet and enjoy!

Nutritional Facts Per Serving:

Calories: 246

Potassium: 139mg

Phosphorus: 217mg

Sodium: 242mg

Protein: 14g

Calcium: 244mg

Carbohydrates: 3g

Fat: 20g

Cholesterol: 237mg

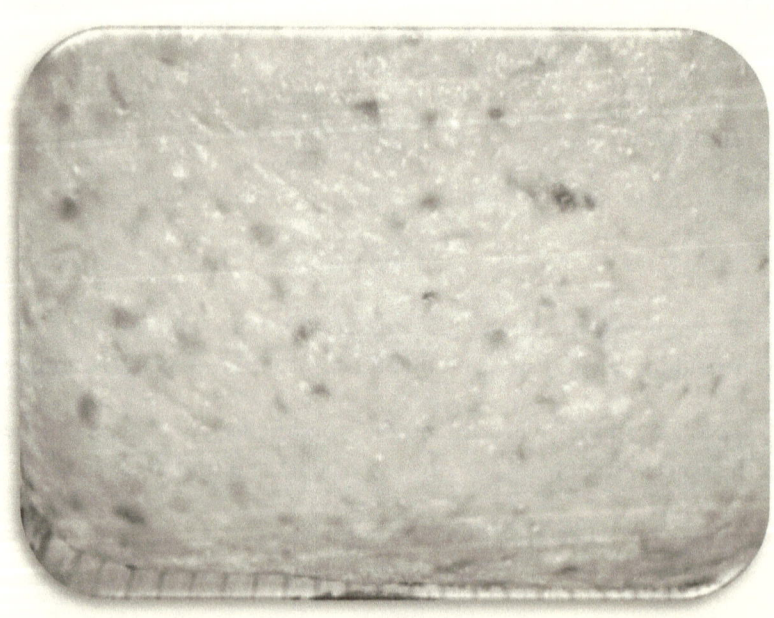

Blueberry Muffins

These freshly baked blueberry muffins makes for a delicious breakfast. Toast Leftover and enjoy later.

Prep Time: 15minutes

Cook Time: 30 minutes

Serves: 12

Ingredients

½ cup unsalted butter

2 eggs

1 ¼ cups sugar

2 cups of milk (1%)

2 cups of all-purpose flour

2 teaspoons of baking powder

2 ½ cups fresh blueberries

½ teaspoon of salt

2 teaspoons sugar

Directions

1. Blend the margarine and sugar in a mixer on low speed, until fluffy. Add one egg, and mix and then add the other until mixed and blended.

2. Sift the dry ingredients, add alternately with milk and then mash and stir ½ cup of blueberries.

3. Spray muffin cups as well as the pan, with oil. Place muffins cups in tin and fill with the muffin mixture. Sprinkle the sugar on top.

4. Place in the oven and bake for about 30 minutes at 375° F. Leave to cool in pan for 45 minutes before carefully removing.

Nutritional Facts Per Serving: 1 serving = 1 muffin

Calories: 275

Potassium: 121 mg

Phosphorus: 100mg

Sodium: 210 mg

Protein: 5g

Calcium: 108 mg

Carbohydrates: 44 g

Fat: 9g

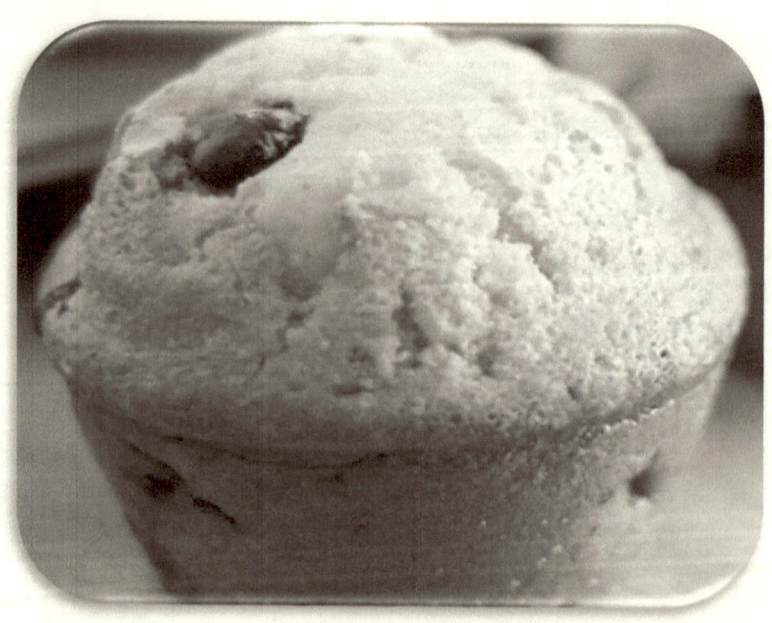

Apple Muffins

Prep Time: 15minutes

Cook Time: 30 minutes

Serves: 12

Ingredients

1 3/4 cups all-purpose flour

1 1/2 teaspoon of baking powder

1/3 cup sugar

1 cup apples, peeled and diced

1/3 cup applesauce, unsweetened

3/4 cup milk, 2%

1/3 teaspoon of ground ginger

1/2 teaspoon of ground cinnamon

Directions

1. Preheat oven to 400°F. Combine the sugar, ginger and cinnamon in a small bowl.

2. In a large bowl, combine the flour, sugar mixture, baking powder, milk and applesauce, beating lightly.

3. Add the sliced apples and stir and then spoon mixture into 12 greased muffin cups.

4. Bake for 20-25 minutes. Let it cool and then serve.

Nutritional Facts Per Serving: 1 serving = 1 muffin

Calories: 105

Potassium: 125mg

Phosphorus: 81mg

Sodium: 10 mg

Protein: 3g

Calcium: 108mg

Carbohydrates: 23g

Simple Baked Pancakes

Prep Time: 15minutes

Cook Time: 20 minutes

Serves: 4

Ingredients

2 large eggs

1/2 cup all-purpose white flour

1/2 cup milk

1/8 teaspoon nutmeg

1/4 teaspoon salt

1 tablespoon vegetable oil

Directions

1. Preheat your oven at 450°F for 5 minutes.

2. In a medium bowl, beat in the eggs and milk in a mixer.

3. Beat in the flour, nutmeg and salt until blended, even if with tiny flour lumps.

4. Pour the oil into a skillet and heat in the oven for 5 minutes.

5. Pour the batter into the skillet and bake, for 20 minutes, uncovered. (Pancake is cooked when the middle is golden brown).

6. Cut into 4 wedges. Enjoy with syrup or fruit spread.

Nutritional Facts Per Serving: 1 wedge or 1/4 recipe

Calories: 189

Potassium: 157mg

Phosphorus: 135mg

Sodium: 206mg

Protein: 8g

Calcium: 90 mg

Carbohydrates: 27g

Fat: 5g

Fruit And Oat Pancakes

Prep Time: 5minutes

Cook Time: 20 minutes

Serves: 4

Ingredients

1 cup flour

1/2 cup of rolled oats

1 8-oz can fruit cocktail, un-drained

1/2 cup liquid non-dairy creamer

1/2 teaspoon baking powder

1 egg

1 tablespoon margarine

Directions:

1. Combine all the ingredients except the margarine in a bowl.

2. In a large skillet, melt the margarine and drop about ¼ cup of batter into the skillet until exhausted. Cover and cook until bubbly.

3. Turn the pancakes over and cook until golden brown.

Nutritional Facts Per Serving: 2 pancakes per serving

Calories: 262

Potassium: 198mg; Phosphorus: 186mg; Sodium: 152mg

Protein: 7g; Calcium: 90 mg; Carbohydrates: 41g; Fat: 8g

TexMex Egg & Tortilla

Enjoy this flavorful scrambled egg for breakfast and do your kidney a lot of good!

Prep Time: 15minutes

Cook Time: 20 minutes

Serves: 6

Ingredients

8 eggs, beaten well

2 green onions, sliced thinly

1 teaspoon chili powder

1/4 cup low sodium ketchup

2 tablespoons of butter

1 bag (6oz) unsalted tortilla chips, broken

Directions

1. Add the chili powder, ketch p and onion to the beaten egg in a bowl and beat until blended.

2. Add the butter to a skillet to melt and then add the tortilla chips. Sauté over medium heat until warm.

3. Add the egg mixture, stir and scramble on desired consistency. Serve!

Buttermilk Pancakes

Prep Time: 10minutes

Cook Time: 20minutes

Serves: 9

Ingredients

2 cups all-purpose flour

1½ teaspoons baking soda

1 teaspoon cream of tartar

2 tablespoons sugar

2 large eggs

2 cups low-fat buttermilk

¼ cup canola oil

Directions

1. In a large bowl, add all the dry ingredients together.

2. In a separate bowl, add all the wet ingredients together.

3. Add the dry and wet ingredients together, whisking with a spoon to blend in the dry ingredients until thoroughly moist.

4. Scoop mixture onto a lightly greased skillet.

5. Cook for a few minutes and then flip with a spatula.

6. Remove to a dish.

Nutritional Facts Per Serving: 2 4-inch pancakes per serving

Calories: 217

Potassium: 182mg; Phosphorus: 100mg; Sodium: 330mg

Protein: 6g ; Calcium: 74 mg; Carbohydrates: 27g; Fat: 9g

Cholesterol: 44 mg

Baked Apple Oatmeal

Prep Time: 12minutes

Cook Time: 15 minutes

Serves: 2

Ingredients

2 tablespoons of cheddar cheese, shredded

1 apple, peeled, cored & sliced thinly

3/4 cup of sweet onion

1/8 teaspoon of black pepper

1 tablespoon of butter

1/4 cup of low fat 1% milk

3 large eggs

Directions

1. Preheat your oven to 400°F

2. Combine milk, eggs, water and milk in a bowl. Mix well.

3. Melt the butter in a pan over medium heat. Add the sliced apple and onion and cook for 5 minutes. Remove once onion is tender.

4. Spread the apple mixture evenly in the pan and then add the egg& milk mixture, spreading and cooking until the edges begin to set. Sprinkle cheddar cheese over.

5. Now place in the oven and bake for 10 minutes and remove once the center is set.

6. Divide into two and enjoy!

Nutritional Facts Per Serving: Calories: 284

Potassium: 341mg; Phosphorus: 238mg; Sodium: 169mg

Protein: 13g; Calcium: 284mg; Carbohydrates: 22g

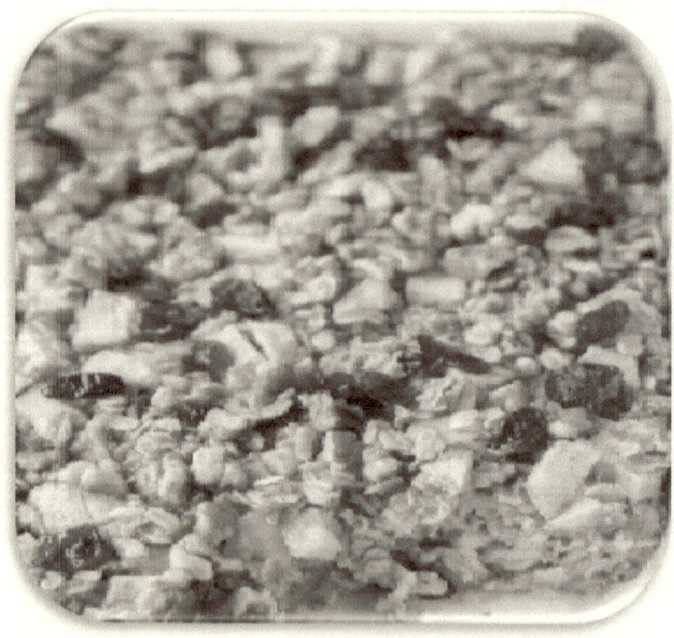

Multigrain Breakfast Cereal

Prep Time: 10minutes

Cook Time: 35 minutes

Serves: 2

Ingredients

1-3/4 cups water

2 tablespoons grits, uncooked

1 tablespoon of whole buckwheat, roasted& uncooked

1 tablespoon of raw bulgur

3 tablespoons of plain raw couscous

1 tablespoon of raw steel-cut oats

Directions

1. Boil water in pot. Add the grits and stir, and then add the buckwheat, bulgur and oats.

2. Stir for a short while and then lower heat to simmer. Spray cooking spray generously on the simmering surface, cover and let it simmer for 25 minutes.

3. Remove from burner; add the couscous and stir. Let it cool for 8 minutes, covered.

4. If desired, top with honey or sweetener of choice. Serve!

Nutritional Facts Per Serving: serving size: 3/4 cup

Calories: 150 kcals

Potassium: 87mg; Phosphorus: 91mg; Sodium: 7mg

Protein: 5g; Calcium: 15 mg; Carbohydrates: 30g

Fat: 1g; Cholesterol: 0 mg

Bran Muffins

Prep Time: 10minutes

Cook Time: 20minutes

Serves: 12

Ingredients

¼ cup of canola oil

1 egg

1 teaspoon of vanilla extract

1/3 cup of honey

1 cup of applesauce, unsweetened

1 cup of wheat bran

1 cup all-purpose flour

1½ teaspoon baking soda

¼ teaspoon cream of tartar

Directions

1. Preheat your oven to 400°F. Grease muffin tins lightly.

2. Combine the egg, applesauce, honey, vanilla and oil together.

3. Add to the mixture, wheat bran, flour, cream of tartar and baking soda. Combine well.

4. Spoon into muffin tins, bake for 20 minutes. Let it cool and then serve.

Nutritional Facts Per Serving:

Calories: 155kcals

Potassium: 126mg

Phosphorus: 100 mg

Sodium: 183mg

Protein: 4g

Calcium: 86mg

Carbohydrates: 21g

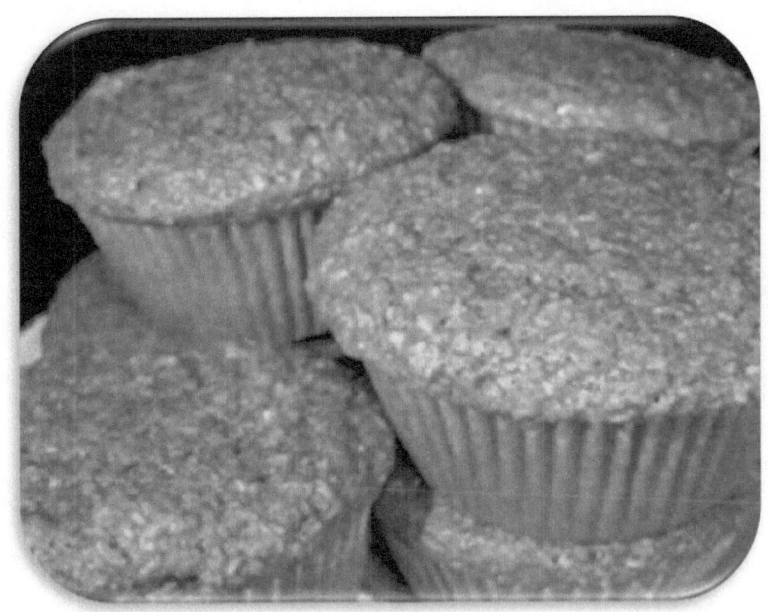

LUNCH

Lunch is an important meal of the day because of the energy it provides to carry on with mental and physical task effectively. People who skip lunch tend to gain more weight because they tend to overeat during dinner to make up for the lost lunch. Since a healthy lunch is good for continuous daily activities, it is important that the lunch you take or pack are low in sodium, potassium and phosphorus and generally ideal for your dietary needs.

If undergoing dialysis, it's good to pack your lunch with you, instead of skipping them, or making do with fast foods or foods from the cafeteria. Anywhere you go, for that matter, it is always safe to have your renal-friendly lunch with you. For instance, pack a renal-friendly healthy sandwich that includes roast beef, turkey, chicken, egg salad or tuna; white bread, pita, bagel tortilla or hamburger buns as well as horseradish and mayonnaise. Do not forget to pack your phosphate binders as well.

Besides sandwiches, there are other delicious and nourishing lunch renal recipes that you can prepare and enjoy at home, work or school. They include, salads such as chicken and rice salads, chicken dishes such as chicken tikka and chicken cutlets, seafood like pan- fried stuffed fish; couscous and vegetable meals you'd love to try.

Sandwiches & Burgers

Parsley Burger

Prep Time: 10minutes

Cook Time: 15minutes

Serves: 4

Ingredients

1 pound lean ground beef or ground turkey

1 tablespoon parsley flakes

1 tablespoon lemon juice

¼ teaspoon ground thyme

¼ teaspoon black pepper

¼ teaspoon oregano

Directions

1. Combine all the ingredients and mix thoroughly.

2. Shape into 4 patties of about ¾" thickness.

3. Grease a skillet or a broiler pan lightly and arrange the patties well on it.

4. Broil 10-15 minutes, ensuring that is about 3" inches from the heat source, turn over once.

Nutritional Facts Per Serving: Serving size: 1 patty, 3-ounces

Calories: 171kcals

Potassium: 289 mg

Phosphorus: 180 mg

Sodium: 108mg

Protein: 20g

Calcium: 21 mg

Carbohydrates: 0 g

Fat: 10g

Cholesterol: 90mg

Couscous Patties

Prep Time: 30 minutes

Cook Time: 20 minutes

Serves: 2

<u>Ingredients</u>

1 cup water

1 cup couscous

1 onion, chopped finely

2 tablespoons extra virgin olive oil

1 clove garlic, crushed

1 celery stalk, chopped finely

½ red capsicum, diced finely

2 teaspoons ground coriander

2 teaspoons ground cumin

2 tablespoons chopped fresh parsley

2 teaspoons lemon rind, grated

2 teaspoons lemon juice

1 egg, beaten lightly

Extra virgin olive oil

For the garden salad:

1 cup of mixed lettuce

8 slices of cucumber

2 rings of green capsicum

2 tablespoons of shallots

2 tablespoons of Italian dressing, low fat

Directions:

1. Bring 1 cup of water to a boil. Pour over the couscous in a bowl and let it stay for 10 minutes. Use a fork to fluff the grains and set aside.

2. Add oil to a pan and cook the onion, capsicum, garlic, celery, ground coriander and cumin until soft.

3. Add the cooked vegetables to the couscous in a bowl and add the lemon rind as well as the fresh parsley, egg and juice. Mix thoroughly.

4. Divide into 4 even portions and shape into large patties. Cover and chill 10 minutes.

5. Cook patties in a little olive oil for 5 minutes per side until golden. Serve with the garden salad.

Nutritional Facts Per Serving: 2 patties with garden salad

Calories: 675kcals

Potassium: 445mg

Phosphorus: 240mg

Sodium: 295mg

Protein: 17g

Carbohydrates: 80g

Fat: 31g

Chicken Burgers

Prep Time: 60minutes

Cook Time: 30minutes

Serves: 4

Ingredients

11½ oz. chicken meat, ground

4oz breadcrumbs

1 medium onion, finely diced

1 teaspoon Dijon mustard

Juice of ½ lemon

1 teaspoon fresh thyme, finely chopped

1 tablespoon olive oil

1 teaspoon, freshly ground black pepper

4 burger buns

For garnish (per burger):

1 slice of tomato

1 slice of red onion

2 slices of cucumber

3 lettuce leaves

¾ tablespoon of mayonnaise

1 teaspoon of Dijon mustard

Directions

1. Combine the chicken, onion, breadcrumbs, mustard, thyme and lemon juice in a large bowl.

2. Season with black pepper and shape into 4 equal patties.

3. Cover and chill 1 hour.

4. Fry in a little olive oil until browned on both sides.

5. Transfer to a pre-heated oven 356° F for 20 minutes.

6. Slice burger buns and toast lightly and then place the patties in the bread

7. Wash the garnish ingredients well, and garnish the burgers.

Nutritional Facts Per Serving: Serving size: 1 patty, 3-ounces

Calories: 480kcals

Potassium: 621 mg; Phosphorus: 346 mg

Protein: 30g; Calcium: 21 mg; Carbohydrates: 50 g

Fat: 19g; Cholesterol: 90mg; Salt: 1.7g

Chili Grilled Cheese Sandwich

Prep Time: 15minutes

Cook Time: 15 minutes

Serves: 4

Ingredients

8 slices of bread

2 tablespoons softened butter or margarine

8 oz. natural Swiss cheese

14-oz can of whole green chilies

Directions

1. Rinse the whole green chilies, split and seed and then open flat.

2. Spread a light portion of margarine or butter on one side of each of the bread.

3. On the plain side of the bread, place an ounce of Swiss cheese and one whole split chili.

4. Now place another ounce of cheese on the split chili and top with the remaining bread slice. Lightly spread the margarine or butter on the bread piece.

5. Place your skillet on medium heat and once hot, place the sandwiches in it and cook, covered on each side until the cheese is melted and the bread is golden brown.

Nutritional Facts Per Serving: Calories: 400 kcals

Potassium: 158mg

Phosphorus: 391mg

Sodium: 267mg

Protein: 20g

Calcium: 603 mg

Carbohydrates: 27g

Fat: 23g

Cholesterol: 52mg

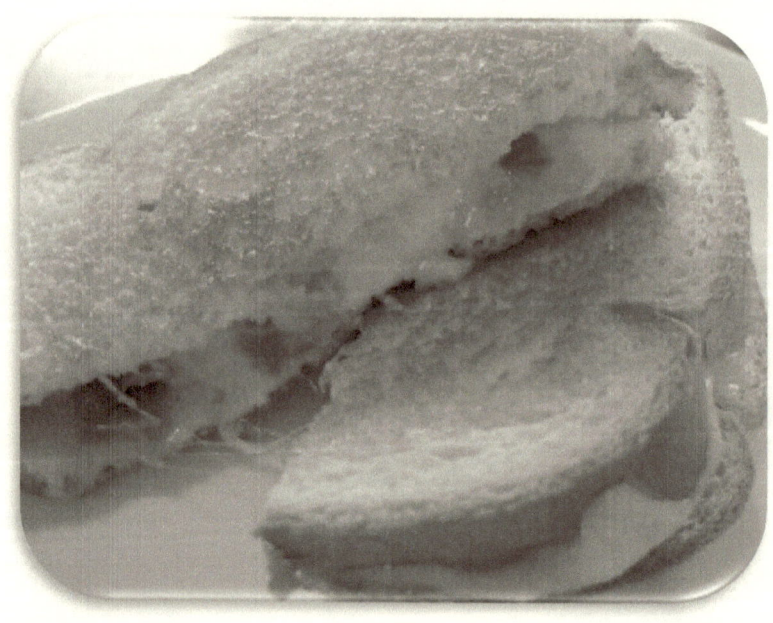

Herb Beef Patties

Prep Time: 2minutes

Cook Time: 10 minutes

Serves: 4

Ingredients

1b lean ground beef

1 teaspoon chopped parsley

1 tablespoon lemon juice

1/4 teaspoon ground thyme

1/4 teaspoon crushed rosemary leaves

Directions

1. Combine all the ingredients thoroughly.

2. Shape mixture into 4 patties very firmly. Place on a grill or on a hot skillet and cook until the center is brown. As the meat cooks, scoop out the fat with a spoon.

3. Garnish with green pepper rings

Nutritional Facts Per Serving: Calories: 194 kcals

Potassium: 361 mg; Phosphorus: 176 mg; Sodium: 82mg

Protein: 23 g; Calcium: 3 mg; Carbohydrates: 30 g

Fat: 10g; Cholesterol: 41 mg

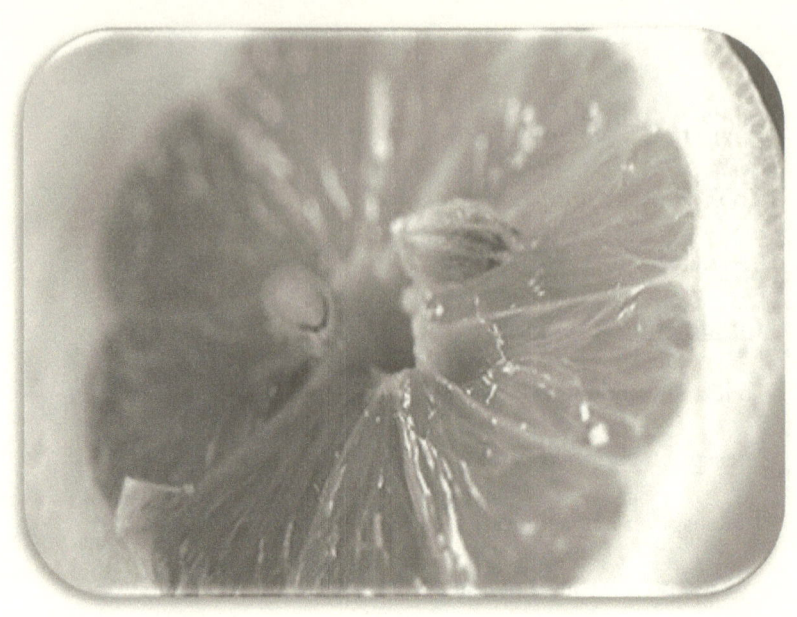

Baked Chicken Broccoli Pizza

Prep Time: 25minutes

Cook Time: 10 minutes

Serves: 4

Ingredients

1 pizza dough, store-bought

2 cups cooked chicken breast, diced

2 cups fresh broccoli florets, blanched

1 cup low-salt mozzarella cheese, shredded

1 tablespoon fresh oregano, chopped

1 tablespoon fresh garlic, chopped

1 teaspoon crushed red pepper flakes

2 tablespoons olive oil

2 tablespoons flour

Directions

1. Begin by preheating your oven to 400°F.

2. In a large bowl, combine the chicken, cheese, broccoli, pepper flakes, oregano and garlic and set aside.

3. Roll out dough on a flour- dusted tabletop until a rectangular shaped dough of about 11" x 14" is formed.

4. Place the chicken mixture close to the edge of the dough (about 2"), along the longest side and then roll, pinch ends and seam them tightly. Brush the top with olive oil and then make 3 small cuts on it.

5. Place in the oven and bake for about 10 minutes until golden brown.

6. Remove. Set aside for a few minutes. Slice and serve.

Nutritional Facts Per Serving: Calories: 522 kcals

Potassium: 546mg

Phosphorus: 400mg

Sodium: 607mg

Calcium: 262mg

Protein: 38 g

Carbohydrates: 52g

Cholesterol: 73mg

Fat: 17g

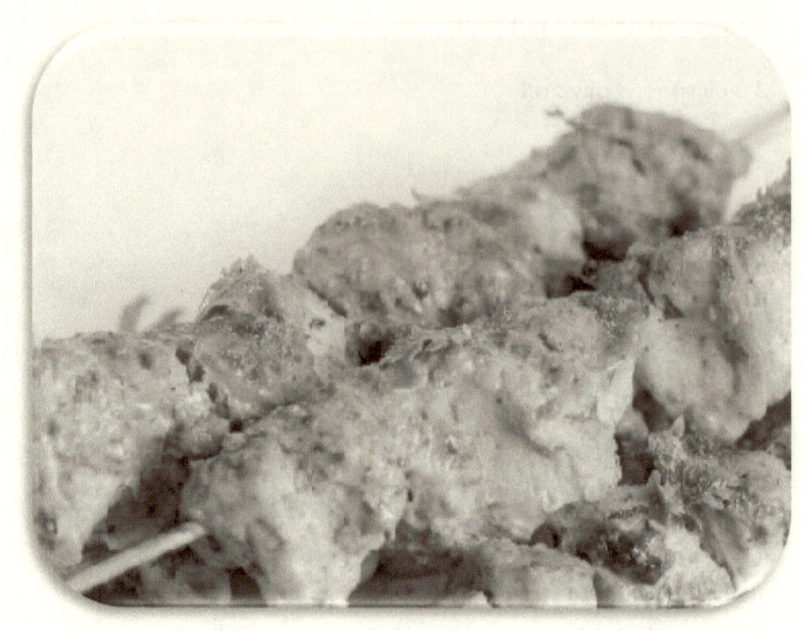

Chicken tikka

Chicken Dishes

Chicken Tikka
A quick, fragrant meal!

Prep Time: 1 hr. 10 minutes

Cook Time: 20minutes

Serves: 2

Ingredients

3 tablespoons of natural yoghurt, low fat

1 teaspoon lemon juice

1 tablespoon curry paste

2 small boneless chicken breasts, skin removed

Directions:

1. Combine the curry paste and yoghurt in a bowl.

2. Drizzle the chicken with the lemon juice and the curried yoghurt.

3. Place in the refrigerator for an hour, at least, or overnight.

4. Place the chicken under a preheated grill and cook for 20 minutes.

5. Serve with boiled rice.

Chicken Schnitzel & Rice Cutlets

Prep Time: 1 hr. 15minutes

Cook Time: 5 minutes

Serves: 6

Ingredients

2 tablespoons of white whole wheat flour

1 teaspoon dry mustard

1/4 cup water

6 pieces of chicken breast cutlets

1/4 teaspoon ground black pepper

1 large raw whole egg

2 large raw egg white

5 ounce of puffed rice

1/2 cup of canola oil

Juice of 1 fresh lemon

Directions

1. Soak the chicken breasts in the lemon juice for an hour. Rinse afterwards, and pat dry.

2. Place the puffed rice in a food processor and crush to bread crumb sizes.

3. Combine the flour and black pepper in a bowl. In another, add together the eggs, mustard powder and water. Place the crushed puffed rice in a third bowl.

4. Coat the chicken breast with flour completely, shaking off excess flour. Dip in egg mixture and then dip again in the puffed rice. Pat to coat evenly and then dip the coated meat back into the egg mixture yet again. Dip in puffed rice as well and pat to coat evenly.

5. Now add the canola oil to a skillet and heat on medium heat. Place in the coated cutlets and cook for a minute. Flip and fry for another minute.

Nutritional Facts Per Serving: Serving Size: 1 cutlet

Calories: 382.18 kcals; Potassium: 318.43 mg; Phosphorus: 18.94mg

Sodium: 260mg; Protein: 26 g; Calcium: 5.9 mg

Carbohydrates: 22g; Fat: 22.54 g; Cholesterol: 86 mg

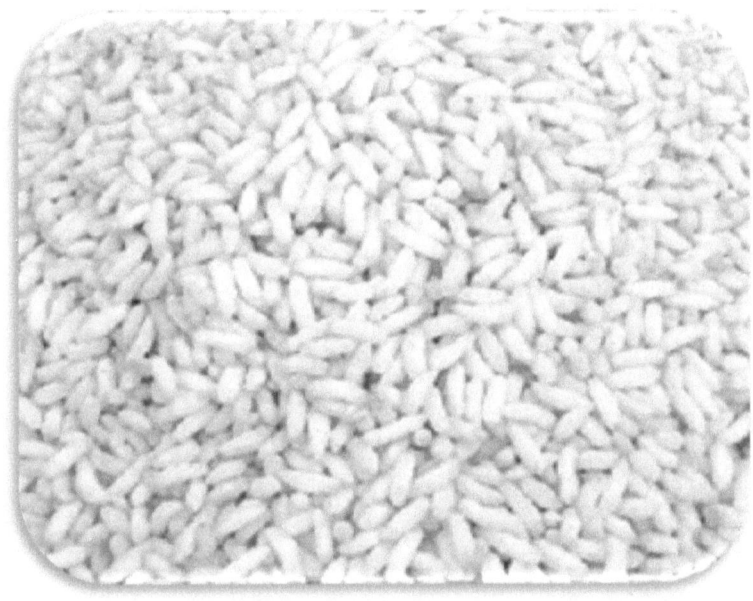

Spicy Curried Chicken

Prep Time: 15minutes

Cook Time: 60 minutes

Serves: 6

Ingredients

1/4 cup olive oil

12 chicken drumsticks

1/2 teaspoon black pepper

1 cup of diced bell pepper, red or yellow

3/4 cup onion, cubed

2 tablespoons fresh ginger, grated

2 cloves garlic, chopped

2 tablespoons Madras curry paste

1 can (14oz) peaches, juice inclusive, diced

3/4 cup plain yogurt

1/4 cup coconut milk

2 tablespoons lime juice

Freshly chopped coriander

Directions

1. Season the drumsticks with pepper all over.

2. Heat the oil in a large skillet and brown the seasoned chicken on medium heat on both sides. Remove chicken.

3. Lower heat and then add the ginger, garlic and curry paste to the pan. Add the onion and pepper and stir to coat thoroughly.

4. Place the chicken back in the pan. Add the peaches with juice. Raise the heat and let it simmer.

5. Cover and place in the oven to cook for 40 minutes at a temperature of 350° F. Remove and place on a stove top set on low heat.

6. Add coconut milk, lime juice and yogurt. Stir until heated through, but do not boil.

7. Serve, garnished with the chopped coriander. Enjoy with white rice.

Nutritional Facts Per Serving: 2 drumsticks

Calories: 406 kcals

Potassium: 519 mg

Phosphorus: 259mg

Sodium: 276mg

Protein: 25 g

Calcium: 30 mg

Carbohydrates: 11g

Fat: 28 g

Cholesterol: 106mg

Chicken Noodle Pancakes

Prep Time: 15 minutes

Cook Time: 30 minutes

Serves: 4

Ingredients

11/2 ounce dry noodles, vermicelli or cellophane

3 eggs

¼ cup plain flour

7 ounce cooked chicken breast, sliced finely

½ cup corn kernels (no added salt)

½ cup green peas or zucchini, grated

2 tablespoons chives, chopped

¼ cup coriander leaves

2 teaspoons low salt soy sauce

1 tablespoon olive

2 tablespoons plum sauce

¼ cup sherry

2 teaspoons reduced salt soy sauce

Directions

1. In a saucepan, add together the plum sauce, sherry and 2 teaspoons of low salt soy sauce and bring to the boil. Keep this glaze warm.

2. Place noodles in a bowl of hot water and leave until soft. Drain and cut into ½ inch lengths.

3. Beat the eggs in a large bowl, and then fold in the flour. Add the chicken, noodles, corn, peas/ zucchini, herbs and soy sauce.

4. Heat a lightly greased non- stick pan over medium heat and pour ¼ of the mixture into the pan.

5. Cook until browned under and egg is set above. Flip egg and brush with the glaze until the other side is cooked as well.

6. Repeat with the rest of the mixture.

7. Spoon extra glaze over each pancake and enjoy.

Nutritional Facts Per Serving: serving size 1 cup

Calories: 310.7 kcals

Potassium: 260mg

Phosphorus: 230mg

Sodium: 405mg

Protein: 20g

Carbohydrates: 24g

Fat: 12g

Seafood Dishes

Herb Topped Fish

Prep Time: 10minutes

Cook Time: 20minutes

Serves: 8

Ingredients

8 (24 oz.) salmon, cut into pieces of 1-1/2 inch thickness

1/2 cup sour cream

1/2 cup mayonnaise

1/4 cup Parmesan cheese, grated

2 tablespoons parsley, chopped

4 tablespoons chives, chopped

1/2 teaspoon dried dill

1/2 teaspoon onion powder

1/2 teaspoon dry mustard

Fresh ground pepper

Directions:

1. Lightly butter a baking pan and place in the uncooked salmon fillets.

2. Blend the rest of the ingredients by hand and sprinkle over the fillets.

3. Bake 20 minutes at a temperature of at 350°F or until fish flakes.

Nutritional Facts Per Serving: 3 ounces per serving

Calories: 244kcals

Potassium: 316 mg

Phosphorus: 239mg

Sodium: 202mg

Protein: 19g

Carbohydrates: 1g

Fat: 18g

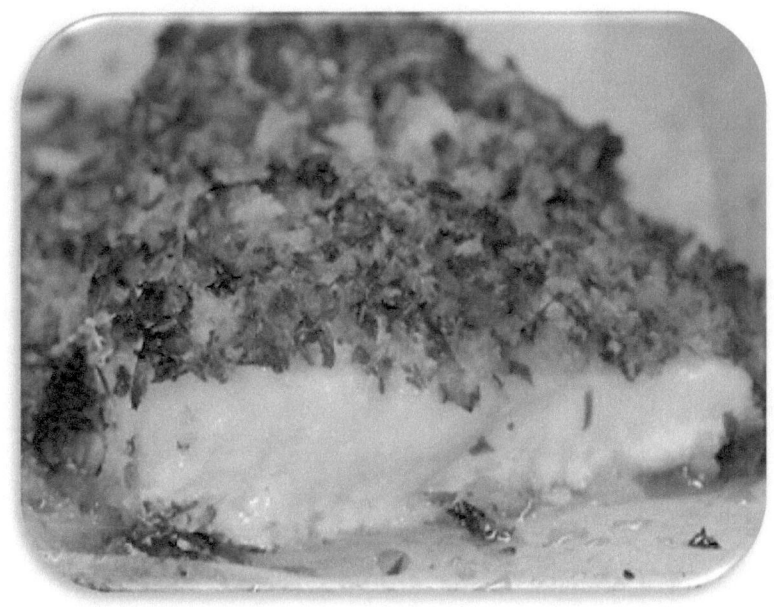

Baked lemon & Paprika Halibut

Prep Time: 5minutes

Cook Time: 15 minutes

Serves: 7

Ingredients

1 1/2 lb. halibut steaks, cut into pieces

3/4 cup bread crumbs

1/4 cup mayonnaise

Lemon slices

Paprika

Directions:

1. Preheat your oven to 400°F.

2. Cover the steak with the mayonnaise completely. Roll in the breadcrumbs and placed in greased or buttered baking pan.

3. Bake 10-15minutes. Serve on heated platter and garnish platter with lemon slices that's been dipped in paprika.

Nutritional Facts Per Serving: 3 ounces per serving

Calories: 205 kcals

Potassium: 456mg; Phosphorus: 233mg; Sodium: 176mg

Protein: 22g; Carbohydrates: 8g; Fat: 9g

White Thatched Cod

Prep Time: 15minutes

Cook Time: 35 minutes

Serves: 4

Ingredients

½ oz. margarine

1oz low fat mayonnaise

4 (18oz) cod fillets

1 small, 4oz onion, chopped

2oz white bread crumbs

1 teaspoon parsley, chopped

Juice and rind of 1 lemon

Directions

1. Melt the margarine in a pan.

2. Place the fillets in a lightly-greased oven proof dish. Arrange in a single layer and brush with a little mayonnaise.

3. Lightly fry the onion in the melted margarine in the pan and add the bread crumbs, lemon rind and juice as well as the parsley.

4. Spoon over the filets in the dish.

5. Cover and bake for 30 minutes at a temperature of 375°F.

Nutritional Facts Per Serving:

Calories: 163 kcals

Potassium: 472mg

Phosphorus: 235mg

Protein: 25.5g

Carbohydrates:8g;

Fat: 3g

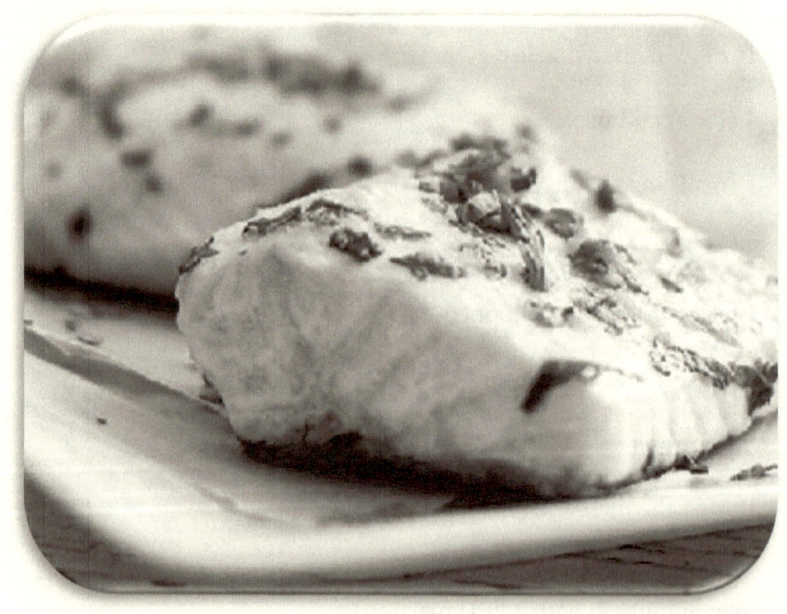

Baked halibut

Tuna Delight

Prep Time: 15minutes

Cook Time: 10 minutes

Serves: 6

Ingredients

1 6-12 ounce can of tuna (rinsed & drained)

1 cup of pineapple chunks, in own natural juice, & drained

1/4 cup green onion, sliced

1/2 cup white rice, cooked and cooled

1/2 cup green peas, cooked & cooled

3/4 cup celery, sliced diagonally

2 tablespoons of lemon juice

1/3 cup of light mayonnaise

Directions

1. Flake the tuna in a medium bowl.

2. In a separate small bowl, combine the mayonnaise and the lemon juice together and mix until smooth. Set aside.

3. Add the rest of the ingredients to the flaked tuna in a bowl. Toss lightly to combine well.

4. Now pour the lemon- mayonnaise mixture into the medium bowl. Stir to blend well. Chill thoroughly, serve with crackers. Garnish with parsley sprig or with fresh mint.

Nutritional Facts Per Serving: 1 cup (1/4 of recipe)

Calories: 195 kcals

Potassium: 340mg

Phosphorus: 116mg

Sodium: 182mg

Protein: 14g

Carbohydrates: 18g

Fat: 7g

Cholesterol: 20

Pan Fried Stuffed Fish

Prep Time: 10minutes

Cook Time: 10 minutes

Serves: 4

Ingredients

1pc (10.5 -14oz) yellow tail fish

2 water chestnuts, chopped finely

2 tablespoons spring onions, diced

2 teaspoons of garlic, chopped

A dash of salt

1 teaspoon of corn flour

A dash of Sesame oil

A dash of pepper powder

Directions

1. To begin, remove the meat from the fish and place in a bowl. Add the sesame oil, pepper powder, salt and corn flour to it and stir to form a paste.

2. Add chestnuts, chopped garlic and spring onions to the paste and mix with hands. This way, any bones in it can be removed easily.

3. Add 2 teaspoons of water to the paste to thicken, if desired.

4. Stuff the paste back into the reserved fish skin and coat the stuffed fish with corn flour.

5. Place in a skillet and fry until golden brown.

6. Cut fish into slices and enjoy!

Nutritional Facts Per Serving:

Calories: 95 kcals

Potassium: 357.8 mg

Phosphorus: 149.8mg

Sodium: 63.8mg

Protein: 12.3 g

Calcium: 3 mg

Carbohydrates: 11.3 g

Fat: 0.7g

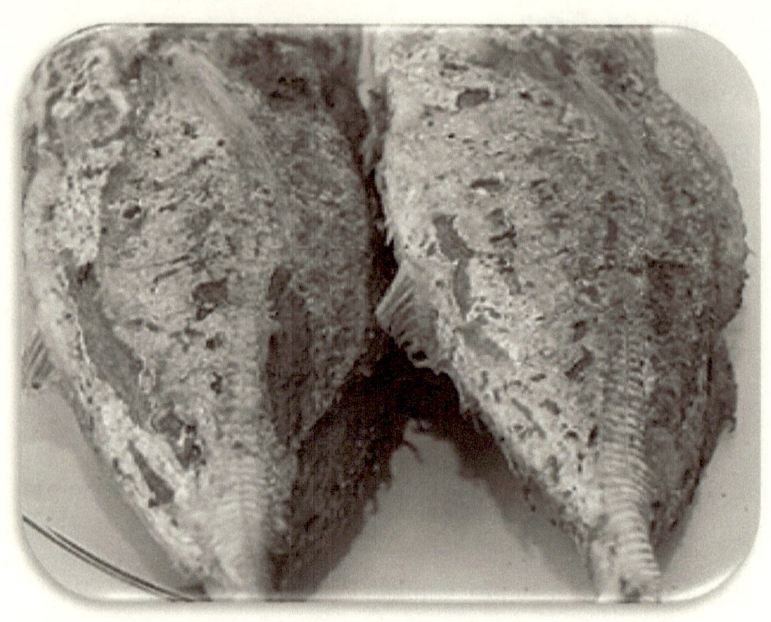

Salmon And Chive Pate

Prep Time: 5 minutes

Cook Time: 0 minutes

Serves: 8

<u>Ingredients</u>

8oz tin salmon, boneless, rinsed & drained

4 oz. cream cheese, softened

5 tablespoons mayonnaise

2 tablespoons lemon juice

2 oz. margarine, melted

2 tablespoons fresh chives, chopped

Directions

1. Add the salmon, mayonnaise, cream cheese, and juice to a blender or food processor and blend to combine well.

2. Add the melted margarine, gradually, and blend to smoothness.

3. Add the chives, stir and pour mixture into ramekins. Chill until set.

4. Enjoy with toast or crackers.

Nutritional Facts Per Serving: Calories: 282 kcals

Potassium: 94 mg; Phosphorus: 63mg; Sodium: 63.8mg

Protein: 6.5 g; Carbohydrates: 0.5 g; Fat: 28g; Salt: 0.7g

Smoky Salmon Dip

Prep Time: 55minutes

Cook Time: 5minutes

Serves:

Ingredients

1 lb. fresh skinless, boneless salmon, cut in pieces of 4

2 cups water

1 cup cream cheese

2 teaspoons smoked paprika

¼ cup capers

¼ cup lemon juice & zest of ½ of a lemon (1 tsp. approx.)

2 tablespoons of red onions, diced finely

1 tablespoon parsley, chopped

1 teaspoon black pepper

Directions

1. Place the salmon, 1 teaspoon of smoked paprika and water in a saucepan or pot, cover and heat for 5 minutes on medium heat. Do not boil.

2. Remove and let it cool for 30- 45 minutes.

3. Combine the rest of the ingredients and mix until smooth.

4. Break the salmon into pieces and fold the pieces into the cream cheese mixture.

5. Let it rest for 30 minutes. Serve with corn chips, celery sticks, and carrots.

Nutritional Facts Per Serving: Calories: 124 kcals

Potassium: 232mg; Phosphorus: 99mg; Sodium: 164mg

Protein: 9g; Carbohydrates: 2g; Fat: 9g; Cholesterol: 42mg

Salad Dishes

Chicken & Rice Salad

Prep Time: 10minutes

Cook Time: 10 minutes

Serves: 6

Ingredients

2 cups cooked rice

21/2 cups cooked chicken, diced

11/2 cups cooked & frozen green peas

1 cup celery, diced

1 tablespoon onion, diced

1/4 light mayonnaise

1/4 cup lemon juice

1/4 teaspoon of pepper

1/8 teaspoon of dill weed

6 large lettuce leaves

Directions

1. Add the rice, chicken together with the onion and celery in a large bowl.

2. In a small bowl, combine the mayonnaise, lemon juice, dill weed and pepper and mix thoroughly.

3. Now mix in the blended mayonnaise mixture into the chicken mixture. Place in the refrigerator for at least 3 hours.

4. Serve salad on lettuce leaf and sprinkle a little paprika over the chicken salad.

Nutritional Facts Per Serving: Calories: 329 kcals

Potassium: 297 mg; Phosphorus: 179 mg; Sodium: 343mg

Protein: 21 g; Calcium: 30 mg; Carbohydrates: 27g

Fat: 15 g; Cholesterol: 62 mg

Summer Pasta Salad

Prep Time: 5minutes

Cook Time: 0 minutes

Serves: 6

Ingredients

2 cups cooked shell macaroni, cooled

1 cup cubed natural yellow cheese, low fat

1 10- ounce package of frozen green peas, cooked, drained & cooled

1/2 cup diced onion

1/8 teaspoon pepper

1/2 teaspoon dried thyme

3/4 cup of light mayonnaise

Directions

1. In a large bowl, add together all the ingredients.

2. Lightly toss together to ensure the mayonnaise blends well with the rest of the ingredients.

3. Add 2 tablespoons of non- dairy creamer or milk to it, if desired.

4. Stir and refrigerate for at least 3 hours or overnight.

Nutritional Facts Per Serving: serving size 1 cup

Calories: 265 kcals; Cholesterol: 14mg

Potassium: 152mg; Phosphorus: 173mg; Sodium: 385mg

Protein: 11g; Calcium: 91 mg; Carbohydrates: 29g; Fat: 11g

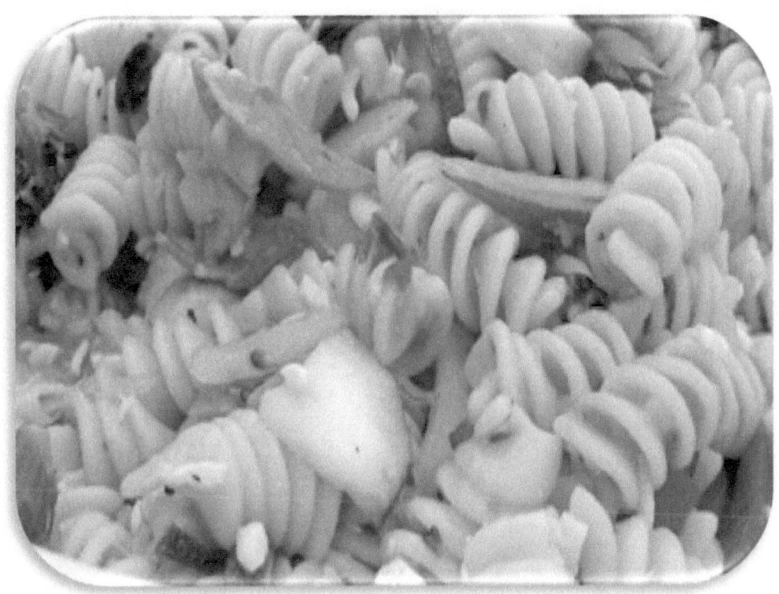

Cranberry Frozen Salad

Prep Time: 10minutes

Cook Time: 0minutes

Serves: 9

Ingredients

1/2 pint whipping cream, whipped

1 8-oz package cream cheese

1/2 teaspoon vanilla extract

1 16-oz can cranberry sauce

Directions:

1. Whip the cream cheese until fluffy.

2. Add in the vanilla, folding in well and then add the whipped cream and then the cranberry sauce.

3. Place in a 9 x 9-inch pan and store in the freezer. Once frozen, cut into squared and serve.

Nutritional Facts Per Serving: Calories: 255 kcals

Potassium: 63mg

Phosphorus: 46mg

Sodium: 99mg

Protein: 2.5g

Carbohydrates: 21g

Fat: 19g

Salmon Salad

Prep Time: 10minutes

Cook Time: 0 minutes

Serves: 1

Ingredients

Small tin of salmon, bones removed

4 round lettuce leaves

1 spring onion

1 handful of watercress

2 beetroot slices

3 red pepper rings

3 new potatoes, halved

1 small tomatoes

1 tablespoon of coleslaw

Directions

1. Boil the potatoes in lots of water until they are soft. Drain afterwards.

2. Add the cut vegetables and toss to mix well.

3, Place the coleslaw and salmon in the middle of the plate and serve.

Macaroni Salad

Prep Time: 10minutes

Cook Time: 0 minutes

Serves: 10

Ingredients

1 lb. elbow macaroni

1/2 cup celery, thinly sliced

1/4 cup sweet onion, diced finely

1 small red sweet bell pepper, diced finely

2 garlic cloves, minced

1 1/2 cups mayonnaise

1 teaspoon apple cider vinegar

2 teaspoons Dijon mustard

1/4 cup sweet pickle relish

1 teaspoon sugar

1/4 teaspoon celery seed

1/2 teaspoon black pepper

3 oz. low-salt bacon, cooked &crumbled

Directions

1. In a large bowl, combine the macaroni, onions, celery and bell pepper together.

2. In a separate bowl, combine the mustard, vinegar, mayonnaise, sugar, pickle relish, celery seed and salt. Stir thoroughly to mix.

3. Stir the salad dressing in to the Macaroni mix. Stir in the crumbled bacon, as well. Enjoy chilled.

Nutritional Facts Per Serving: serving size 1 cup

Calories: 322 kcals

Sodium: 318mg

Protein: 6.5g; Calcium: 91 mg

Carbohydrates: 46.4 g; Fat: 12.6g

Cholesterol: 9.2mg

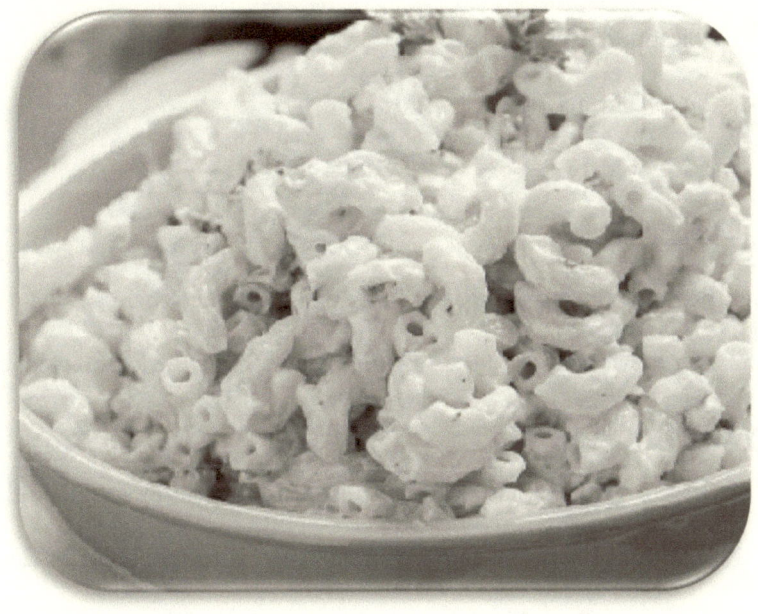

Shrimp Macaroni Salad

Prep Time: 10minutes

Cook Time: 10 minutes

Serves: 4

Ingredients

2 cups of cooked elbow macaroni, cooled (1 cup uncooked)

1 cup cucumber, peeled and diced

8 oz. cooked, baby shrimp, fresh or frozen

1 tablespoon of minced onion

1/4 teaspoon of pepper

1 tablespoon of minced parsley

1/2 cup light mayonnaise

4 lemon wedges

Directions

1. Begin by rinsing the frozen shrimp in cold water, drain and pat dry.

2. In a bowl, add together all the ingredients, save the lemon wedges.

3. Toss to blend ingredients thoroughly with the mayonnaise.

4. Serve on red leaf lettuce and garnish with the lemon wedges and paprika.

Nutritional Facts Per Serving: 1 cup (1/4 of recipe) Calories: 256 kcals

Potassium: 182mg; Phosphorus: 114mg; Sodium: 371mg

Calcium: 34mg; Protein: 17g; Fat: 11g; Cholesterol: 121

Orzo Salad

Prep Time: 5minutes

Cook Time: 10 minutes

Serves: 4

Ingredients

4 cups of cooked orzo, chilled (1 2/3 cup of dried orzo)

1/4 cup of extra-virgin olive oil

1/4 cup of lemon juice

2 cups apple, diced

1/2 teaspoon black pepper, freshly ground

2 tablespoon fresh basil, chopped

1/2 cup crumbled blue cheese

1/4 cup blanched almonds, chopped

Directions

1. Combine all the ingredients, except the almonds and blue cheese, in a bowl. Mix gently to incorporate well.

2. Pour the mixture in a serving dish and sprinkle with the reserved blue cheese and almonds. Serve!

Nutritional Facts Per Serving: 1 cup (1/4 of recipe)

Calories: 276 kcals

Potassium: 153mg; Phosphorus: 52mg; Calcium: 34mg

Protein: 6g; Carbohydrate: 39 g; Fat: 11g; Cholesterol: 6mg

Vegetable Dishes

Super Lunch Bowl

Prep Time: 5minutes

Cook Time: 20 minutes

Serves: 4

Ingredients

2 tablespoons of oil

4 celery stalks, diced

1 red pepper, diced

1 green pepper, diced

2 jalapeno peppers, seeded and diced

½ cup onion, diced

Pinch chili powder

4 springs parsley or cilantro

4 eggs

4 mandarin orange slices

4 small flour tortillas, warmed

Directions

1. Place a large skillet over medium heat and then add the oil and once hot, add the celery, peppers and onion and cook for 15 minutes on medium low heat.

2. Break the eggs, one at a time, on the sautéed veggies. Ensure that the eggs are separate from the others as you crack.

3. Do not scramble or stir but cover the pan for 5 minutes or until the eggs are cooked.

4. To serve, remove the vegetable portion that has an egg on top and place on a plate. Do this for the four plates and then garnish with orange slices.

5. Enjoy as a side with warmed tortillas.

Nutritional Facts Per Serving:

Calories: 277 kcals

Potassium: 403 mg

Phosphorus: 142mg

Sodium: 267mg

Protein: 10 g

Calcium: 94 mg

Carbohydrates: 26g

Fat: 15g

Cholesterol: 212mg

Crispy Fried Okra

Prep Time: 10 minutes

Cook Time: 20 minutes

Serves: 4

Ingredients

1 16-oz package frozen okra, thawed & cut

1/2 cup cornmeal

1/2 cup flour

1/4 teaspoon pepper

2 tablespoons margarine

1 cup water

Directions:

1. Add together the cornmeal, flour and pepper in a bowl.

2. Add in the margarine and mix until crumbly.

3. Dip the okra in water, coat in the cornmeal mixture and place on a lightly greased baking sheet.

4. Bake for 20 minutes at 350°F. Remove once golden brown and enjoy with low- sodium ketchup of choice.

Nutritional Facts Per Serving: 1/2 Cup Per Serving

Calories: 215 kcals

Potassium: 208mg; Phosphorus: 71 mg; Sodium: 56mg

Protein: 4g; Carbohydrates: 36g; Fat: 6g

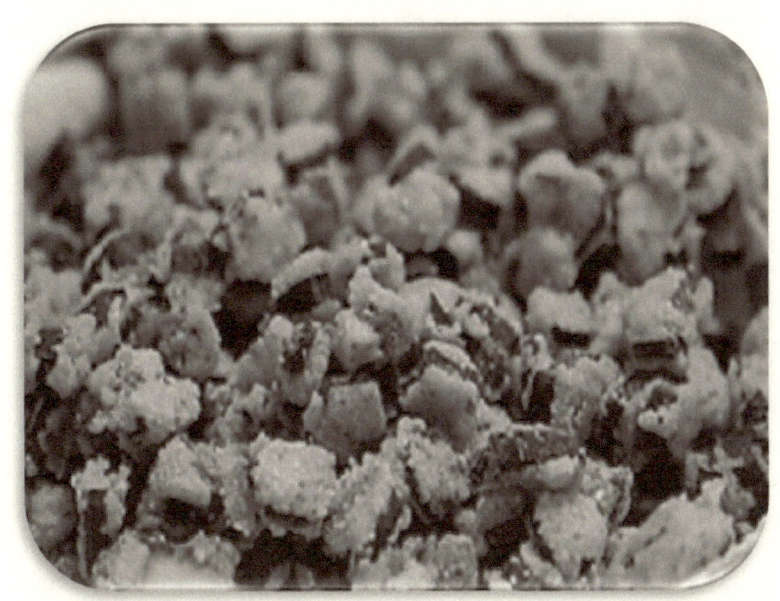

Vegetable Cutlets

Prep Time: 10minutes

Cook Time: 45 minutes

Serves: 6

<u>Ingredients</u>

1 cup of carrots, grated

2 cups of cabbage, grated

2 cups of French beans, chopped

¼ teaspoon salt

1 teaspoon coriander powder

1 teaspoon cumin powder

1 teaspoon red chili powder

½ cup all-purpose flour

4 white slices of bread

¼ cup fresh coriander, chopped

½ teaspoon lime juice

2 tablespoons of vegetable oil

Directions

1 Place the carrots and cabbage in a pan and boil on medium heat. Halfway through cooking, add the French beans and cook until done. Drain water.

2. Add the spices and flour as well as the bread slices, (the bread slices must be soaked in water and squeezed by hand to drain), coriander and lime juice.

3. Next make into balls of 12 and flatten.

4. Place a pan over medium heat and add the oil. Place the patties in the pan, 2 -3 at a time at a time to prevent crowding and cook for 2- 3 minutes. Flip and cook until done.

5. Serve!

Nutritional Facts Per Serving: 2 cutlets

Calories: 145 kcals

Potassium: 241mg; Phosphorus: 60mg; Sodium: 219mg

Protein: 4g; Carbohydrates: 21g; Fat: 5g

Mashed Gingered Carrots

Prep Time: 10 minutes

Cook Time: 0minutes

Serves: 2

Ingredients

½ teaspoon fresh ginger, chopped

2 cups of baby carrots

½ teaspoon black pepper

½ teaspoon honey

½ teaspoon vanilla extract

1 tablespoon fresh chives, chopped

Directions

1. Steam carrots until carrots tender.

2. Set heat to low and mash the steamed carrots.

3. Add the rest of the ingredients, except the chives, and stir to mix well.

4. Serve, garnished with the fresh chives.

Nutritional Facts Per Serving: Calories: 30kcals

Potassium: 174mg; Phosphorus: 21 mg; Sodium: 55mg

Calcium: 25mg; Protein: 1g; Carbohydrates: 7g

Fat: 0g; Cholesterol: 0mg

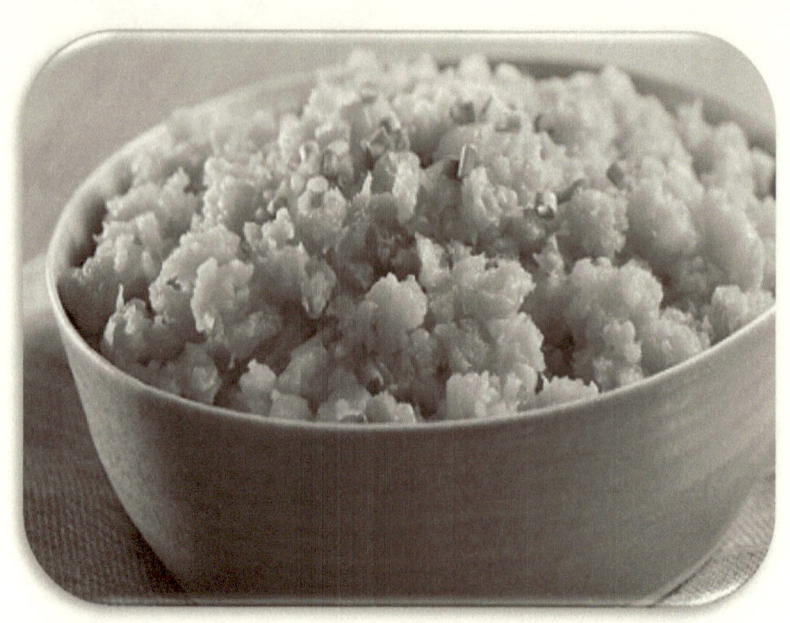

Parmesan & Herb Sautéed Zucchini

Prep Time: 15 minutes

Cook Time: 10 minutes

Serves: 6

<u>Ingredients</u>

3-medium-size zucchini, sliced (4 cups)

½ cup flour

1 cup whole milk

¼ cup Parmesan cheese, grated

½ teaspoon fresh thyme

½ teaspoon fresh basil

2 tablespoons vegetable oil

½ teaspoon fresh tarragon

Pepper to taste

Directions

1. Soak the fresh zucchini in milk.

2. In a bowl, combine the flour, cheese and pepper and then add the herbs.

3. Add the oil to a large pan and heat.

4. Dip the zucchini in parmesan cheese and herb mixture.

5. Finally, sauté in oil and serve hot.

Nutritional Facts Per Serving: Calories: 130kcals

Potassium: 266mg

Phosphorus: 98mg

Sodium: 75mg

Calcium: 97mg

Protein: 4g

Carbohydrates: 12g

Fat: 7g

Cholesterol: 7mg

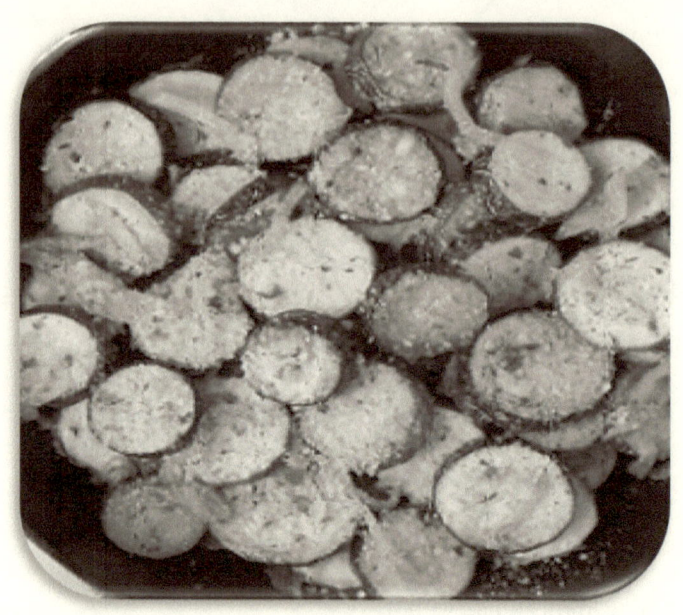

Mediterranean Green Beans
Simply delicious!

Prep Time: 10minutes

Cook Time: 7minutes

Serves: 4

<u>Ingredients</u>

1 lb. fresh green beans, trimmed

¾ cup water

3 fresh garlic cloves, minced

2½ teaspoons olive oil

3 tablespoons of fresh lemon juice

1/8 teaspoon of ground black pepper

Directions

1. Pour the water into a skillet and bring to a boil. Add the beans and cook for 3 minutes. Drain and set to one side.

2. Heat oil in a skillet and add the garlic and the cooked beans. Sauté a minute and then add the juice and the ground black pepper. Sauté a minute longer.

Nutritional Facts Per Serving: Calories: 71kcals

Potassium: 186mg; Phosphorus: 37 mg; Sodium: 2mg

Calcium: 55mg; Protein: 2g; Carbohydrates: 10g

Fat: 3g; Cholesterol: 0mg

Garlic Potato Mash
Prep Time: 20minutes

Cook Time: 10minutes

Serves: 1

Ingredients

9oz potato, boiled

1 large, clove of garlic, crushed

1 tablespoon of natural yoghurt

1 tablespoon of sour cream

Directions

1. Boil and drain the potatoes.

2. Add the garlic, sour cream and yoghurt.

3. Mash and enjoy!

Nutritional Facts Per Serving:

Calories: 193kcals

Potassium: 376mg

Phosphorus: 109mg, Sodium: 0.08mg

Protein: 2g, Carbohydrates: 37g, Fat: 3.7g

Summer Vegetable Sauté
Prep Time: 10minutes

Cook Time: 15minutes

Serves: 6

Ingredients

2 tablespoons margarine

2 cups zucchini, sliced

1/2 cup green pepper, diced

1 10-oz package frozen corn, thawed

2 tablespoons pimiento, chopped

1/8 teaspoon garlic powder

1/8 teaspoon pepper

Directions:

1. In a large pan, heat the margarine and add the rest of the ingredients.

2. Sauté about 15 minutes or until vegetables are tender.

Nutritional Facts Per Serving:

Calories: 81kcals

Potassium: 175mg

Phosphorus: 38mg

Sodium: 38mg

Protein: 2g

Carbohydrates: 9g

Fat: 4g

Quick Chickpea Curry

Prep Time: 10minutes

Cook Time: 15minutes

Serves: 2

Ingredients

2 teaspoons oil

2 cloves garlic, crushed

1 teaspoon of ground ginger powder or fresh ginger, 1 inch, peeled and chopped finely

1 tablespoon curry paste

1 small (8oz) tin chopped tomatoes

6 tablespoons of water

1 onion, peeled and chopped

1 15oz tin chickpeas in water, drained

Handful fresh coriander leaves, chopped

<u>Directions:</u>

1. Fry the garlic, onion, curry paste and ginger in the oil for 2 or 3 minutes.

2. Drain the juice in the tin of tomatoes and discard, and then add the tomatoes, together with the water, and cook for a minute longer.

3. Now add the chickpeas and almost all the coriander and cook for about 10 minutes or until reduced.

4. Add the rest of the coriander and stir to mix.

5. Serve, garnished with spring onions and sliced cucumber sticks. Enjoy with naan bread

Couscous

Moroccan Couscous

Prep Time: 10minutes

Cook Time: 5 minutes

Serves: 4

Ingredients

2 tablespoons of chopped onion

1/2 tablespoon olive oil

2/3 cup dry couscous

1 cup water

Directions:

1. Sauté the onion in the olive oil until translucent.

2. Bring the water to a boil in a saucepan.

3. Add the couscous and onion and stir. Let it rest for 5 minutes.

4. Fluff with fork lightly. Serve!

Nutritional Facts Per Serving: 1/2 Cup Per Serving

Calories: 115 kcals

Potassium: 61 mg

Phosphorus: 22 mg

Sodium: 24mg

Protein: 3.5 g

Calcium: 30 mg

Carbohydrates: 21g

Fat: 2 g

Mint Couscous

Prep Time: 10minutes

Cook Time: 15minutes

Serves: 4

Ingredients

8oz couscous

21/2 cups water

3 tablespoons of fresh mint chopped

2 teaspoons of olive oil

Directions

1. Pour the water into a saucepan and bring to a boil.

2. Remove and add in the couscous; stir and cover. Let it rest for 5 minutes and then fluff with a fork.

3. Add oil and mint, and seasoned as desired.

4. Serve with grilled fish or meat.

Lemon & Coriander Couscous

Prep Time: 10minutes

Cook Time: 15minutes

Serves: 4

Ingredients

8oz couscous

2 1/2 cups water

3 tablespoons of fresh coriander, chopped

Juice and grated rind of 1 lemon

2 teaspoons of olive oil

Directions

1. Pour the water into a saucepan and bring to a boil.

2. Remove and add in the couscous; stir and cover. Let it rest for 5 minutes and then fluff with a fork.

3. Add oil and coriander, as well as the lemon juice and rind.

4. Season with black pepper.

DINNER

Dinner is a very important meal of the day. Besides the opportunity of deepening bonds when friends and family come together to share a meal, it is also a great health booster. Eating a healthy dinner ensures better sleep because lack of sound overtime can increase the risk of high blood pressure, which can aggravate kidney failure. A healthy dinner also helps to manages weight, boost energy and promotes health.

If you have kidney failure, eating a healthy dinner provides you with accurate amounts of nutrients that is needed for your kidney health. Eat early as well. Below are very delicious and nutritious renal friendly dishes: from chicken, to pork, beef, seafood, vegetables, soups and stews; your choice is endless. You are certain of eating right, sleeping right and promoting your kidney health.

Chicken Dishes

Chicken With Dill & Honey Sauce

Prep Time: 40minutes

Cook Time: 20 minutes

Serves: 4

Ingredients

¾ cup breadcrumbs

2 tablespoons of Parmesan cheese

¼ teaspoon pepper

1 ½ teaspoon dried thyme

¾ teaspoon garlic powder

¾ teaspoon onion powder

½ cup light mayonnaise

¼ cup liquid honey

½ teaspoon dried dill weed

4 chicken breast halves, (boneless & skinless, cut into strips of 1")

¼ cup unsalted margarine, melted

Directions

1. Combine the dill weed, honey and mayonnaise in a bowl, cover and chill for 30 minutes.

2. Next, preheat your oven to 400°F. Add together the breadcrumbs, cheese, thyme, pepper, onion powder and garlic powder.

3. Dip the chicken in the melted margarine and dip again in the breadcrumb mixture to coat.

4. Place on a greased baking rack, bake for 10 minutes and then flip and bake for an additional 10 minutes.

Nutritional Facts Per Serving: 3 strips per serving

Calories: 290 kcals

Potassium: 262mg

Phosphorus: 247mg

Sodium: 300mg

Protein: 28 g

Carbohydrates: 15 g

Moroccan Honey Chicken

Prep Time: 5minutes

Cook Time: 40 minutes

Serves: 6

Ingredients

1/3 cup honey

2 tablespoons lemon juice

1 teaspoon sesame oil

½ teaspoon lemon zest

½ teaspoon ground cumin

3 cloves garlic, crushed

1 teaspoon paprika

¼ teaspoon cinnamon

¼ teaspoon of onion powder

¼ teaspoon nutmeg

¼ teaspoon black pepper

½ teaspoon pepper, cayenne

6 chicken thighs or breast, bone in, no skin

Directions

1. Combine all the ingredients, save the chicken, in a bowl.

2. Now, add the chicken to marinate and chill for several hours or overnight.

3. Place chicken on lined baking sheet with the bone down and spoon extra marinade over it.

4. Bake for 30 to 40 minutes at a temperature of 400°F.

5. Enjoy with rice or couscous.

Nutritional Facts Per Serving: 1 chicken thigh

Calories: 196kcals

Potassium: 305mg; Phosphorus: 218mg; Sodium: 79mg

Protein: 26g; Carbohydrates: 16g; Fat: 3g

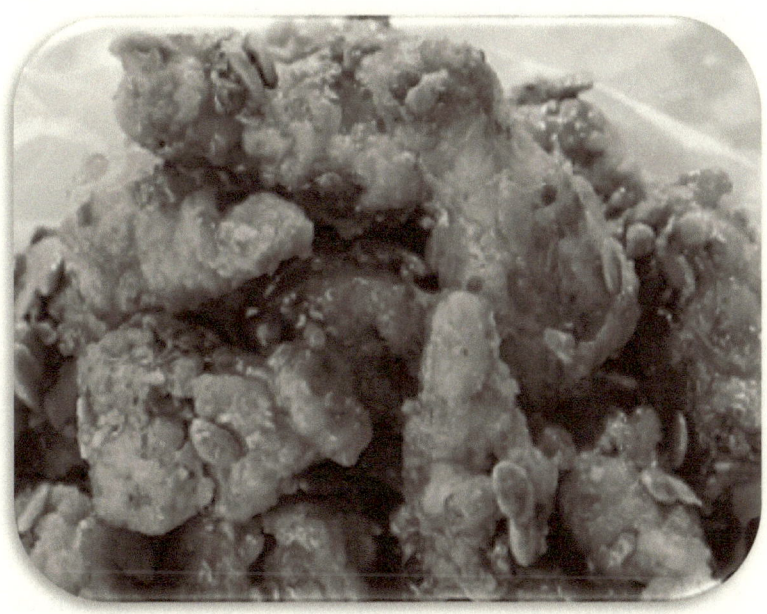

Chicken Stew

Prep Time: 10minutes

Cook Time: 35minutes

Serves: 6

Ingredients

3 tablespoon vegetable oil

2 lb. chicken breast, cut into pieces

1 cup onions, sliced

2 cloves garlic, minced

¾ cup green peppers

2 tablespoon all-purpose flour

2 10 ½-ounce cans chicken broth, low-sodium

1 10-ounce bag frozen carrots

¼ teaspoon black pepper

¼ teaspoon dried basil

1 110-ounce bag frozen sliced okra

Directions

1. In a Dutch oven, add in 2 tablespoons of oil and the chicken and sauté over medium high heat.

2. Once the chicken is browned, remove and set aside. Add the 1 tablespoon of oil that's left and sauté the onion, garlic and pepper.

3. Add flour and cook with constant stirring. Add the chicken and broth and keep cooking until boiling.

4. Now add the carrots and basil as well as the black pepper. Cover and let it simmer for 10 minutes to thicken.

5. Add okra, cook 5-10 more minutes. Enjoy with hot white rice.

Nutritional Facts Per Serving: Serving size: 1 cup

Calories: 142 kcals

Potassium: 453mg; Phosphorus: 129mg; Sodium: 93mg

Calcium: 69mg; Protein: 10g; Carbohydrates: 13g

Fat: 8g; Cholesterol: 15mg

Chicken Mole

Prep Time: 5minutes

Cook Time: 70 minutes

Serves: 12

<u>Ingredients</u>

1 chicken, cut & skinned

1 tablespoon of olive oil

1/2 medium onion, diced

1/2 green pepper, diced

1 garlic clove, crushed

Cayenne pepper to taste

1 tablespoon chili powder

1 tablespoon cocoa

1- 14 ounce can tomatoes, no salt added, drained & diced

3 cups of cooked white rice cooked.

Directions

1. Add oil to a large skillet and sauté the onion, green pepper and garlic.

2. Add the diced tomatoes, cayenne pepper and chili powder. Dilute the cocoa in 2 teaspoons of water and add to the mixture. Stir to combine well.

3. Add the chicken to the skillet. Let it simmer for 1 hour on low heat and then serve with ½ cup of hot rice.

Nutritional Facts Per Serving:

Calories: 321 kcals

Potassium: 447mg

Phosphorus: 365mg

Sodium: 207mg

Calcium: 39mg

Protein: 35 g

Carbohydrates: 27g

Cholesterol: 103

Fat: 7g

Chicken With Mustard Sauce

Prep Time: 25minutes

Cook Time: 20minutes

Serves: 8

Ingredients

2 lb. chicken breast, sliced thinly

¼ cup shallots, diced

¼ cup fresh scallions, chopped

½ cup canola oil

½ cup flour

2 cups low-sodium chicken stock

1 tablespoon low sodium Chicken Base, preferably Bouillon

½ stick of unsalted butter, cubed

2 tablespoons brown mustard

Seasoning ingredients:

½ teaspoon black pepper

½ teaspoon Italian seasoning

1 tablespoon smoked paprika

1 tablespoon dried parsley

Directions

1. In a small bowl, add together the Italian seasoning, parsley, paprika and pepper. Sprinkle half of the mixture on the breasts and add the rest to the flour.

2. Remove 3 tablespoons of the seasoned flour and set to one side. Dredge the chicken in the seasoned flour.

3. In a large skillet, sauté the seasoned and dredged chicken in hot canola oil for 2 minutes per side. Remove to a plate.

4. Remove the oil from the skillet, leaving only 2-3 tablespoons. Sauté the shallots in it until translucent.

5. Now, whisk in the flour until smooth and the stock gradually with constant whisking. Cook on medium heat for 5 minutes and then add the chicken billion, unsalted butter and mustard, whisking to mix.

6. Turn heat off, return chicken with drippings to pan and stir. Serve, garnished with scallions.

Nutritional Facts Per Serving:

Calories: 351 kcals

Potassium: 497mg

Phosphorus: 283mg

Sodium: 393mg

Calcium: 24mg

Protein: 28 g

Carbohydrates: 9g

Cholesterol: 113

Fat: 22g

Chicken Sweetcorn Stir Fry

Prep Time: 10minutes

Cook Time: 25minutes

Serves: 2

Ingredients

7 oz. Chicken breast, cut into strips

2 small shallots, chopped

1 small can of sweetcorn, drained

30g Frozen peas

2 tablespoons of half fat crème fraîche (heaped)

Olive oil

Black pepper

Directions:

1. Add a little oil to a pan, add the shallots and chicken and fry, with frequent stirring, for about 15 minutes or until chicken is browned.

2. Add the sweetcorn and peas and stir and cook for extra minutes.

3. Add the crème fraîche, and season dish with black pepper. Stir thoroughly.

4. Enjoy with boiled rice.

Nutritional Facts Per Serving: without rice

Calories: 390 kcals

Potassium: 21mmol; Phosphorus: 14mmol

Sodium: 18mml; Protein: 36g; Fat: 13g

Chicken And Gnocchi Dumplings
A kidney friendly classic comfort food!

Prep Time: 15minutes

Cook Time: 45 minutes

Serves: 10

Ingredients

2 pounds chicken breast

1 pound store bought gnocchi

¼ cup light olive oil

1 tablespoon low sodium Bouillon Chicken Base

6 cups chicken stock, reduced-sodium

½ cup fresh celery, finely diced

½ cup fresh carrots, finely diced

½ cup fresh onions, finely diced

¼ cup fresh parsley, chopped

1 teaspoon Italian seasoning

1 teaspoon black pepper

Directions

1. In a stockpot, brown the chicken in hot oil on all sides.

2. Add the carrots, onions and celery and cook until translucent. Add the chicken stock cook for 20 to 30 minutes on high heat.

3. Lower heat; add the chicken bouillon, Italian seasoning and black pepper and stir.

4. Finally, add the gnocchi and cook with constant stirring for 15 minutes.

5. Remove from heat; add the parsley. Serve!

Nutritional Facts Per Serving:

Calories: 362 kcals

Potassium: 485mg

Phosphorus: 295mg

Sodium: 121mg

Calcium: 38mg

Protein: 28 g

Carbohydrates: 38g

Cholesterol: 158mg

Fat: 10g

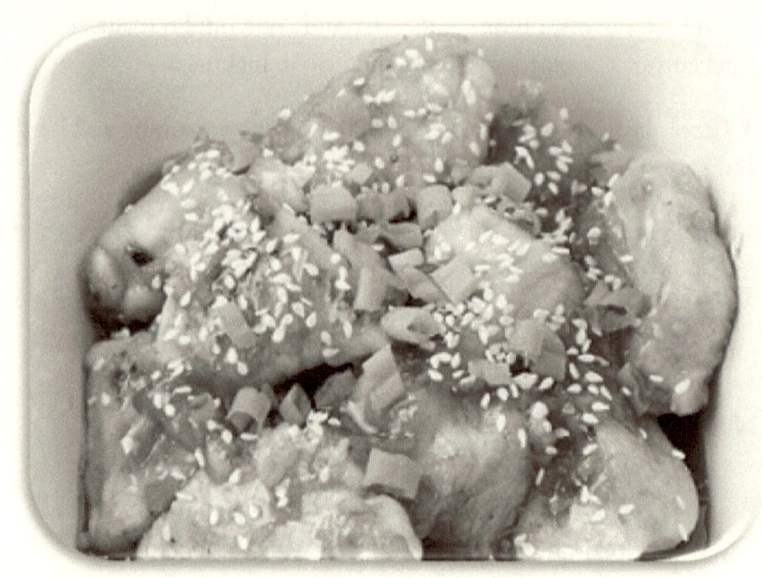

Orange chicken

Chicken With Orange And Ginger

Prep Time: 5minutes

Cook Time: 30 minutes

Serves: 4

Ingredients

4 skinless chicken breasts

1 tablespoon honey

1 tablespoon mustard

Grated rind of 1orange

3 tablespoons orange juice

2 teaspoons of ground ginger powder

Directions

1. Preheat oven to 375°F.

2. Make 3 slits across each piece of chicken and place in a casserole dish.

3. Combine the honey, mustard, ground ginger, orange zest and orange juice.

4. Spoon mixture over the chicken and cook in the oven for about 30 minutes.

5. Serve with boiled rice or new potatoes and desired boiled vegetables.

Chicken Veronique

Prep Time: 10minutes

Cook Time: 30minutes

Serves: 5

Ingredients

1 tablespoon flour

1 lb. chicken breast meat

1/4 teaspoon pepper

6 tablespoons margarine, unsalted

1/2 cup water

1/4 cup white wine

1/4 teaspoon pepper

1 teaspoon parsley

2 tablespoons orange marmalade

1 bay leaf

1 cup halved white grapes

Directions:

1. Add together the flour and 1/4 teaspoon pepper. Sprinkle lightly over the chicken.

2. In a large skillet, sauté the chicken in margarine on all sides until golden brown.

3. Add the rest of the ingredients, save the grapes. Cover and let it simmer for 25 minutes. Chicken should be tender by then.

4. Remove to a platter. To the gravy, add the grapes and cook, with constant stirring for about 2 minutes. Pour over the chicken.

Nutritional Facts Per Serving: Serving size: 2/3 cup

Calories: 275 kcals

Potassium: 284mg

Phosphorus: 179mg

Sodium: 178mg

Calcium: mg

Protein: 22g

Carbohydrates: 13 g

Fat: 15 g

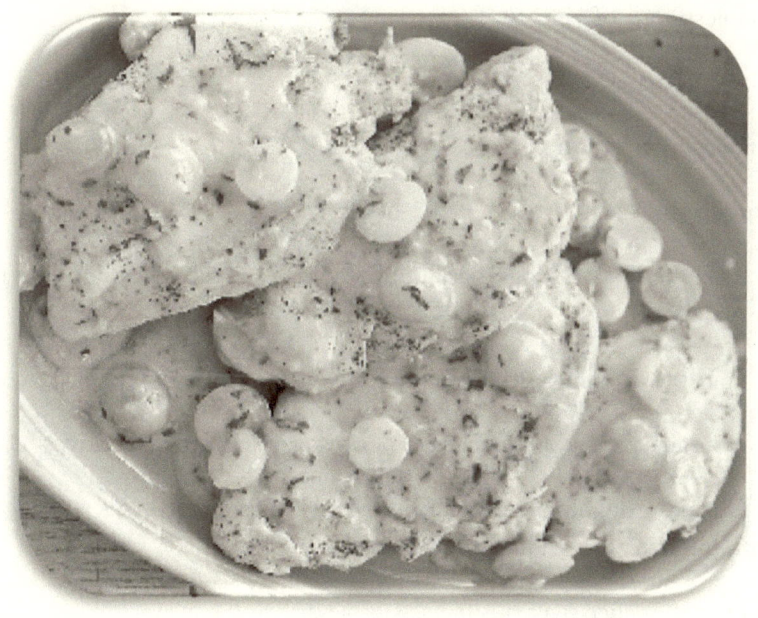

Cranberry Spareribs

Prep Time: 20 minutes

Cook Time: 1 hr. 20 minutes

Serves: 6

Ingredients

3 lbs. spareribs

¼ cup of brown sugar

3 tablespoons of flour

¼ teaspoon of dry mustard

¼ teaspoon of ground cloves

14 oz. can cranberry sauce

2 tablespoons of vinegar

2 cups of water

1 tablespoon lemon juice

Directions

1. Broil the ribs on broiler rack until brown. Turn the other side over to brown as well.

2. Pour the drippings off, rinse the ribs with warm water and place in a dish.

3. In a saucepan, add together the flour, sugar, mustard and cloves.

4. Once thoroughly combined, add the rest of the ingredients and cook, with frequent stir, until quite thickened.

5. Pour the sauce over ribs in a casserole dish and cover.

6. Bake for an hour at a temperature of 350°F. Uncover dish at last 15minutes of cooking.

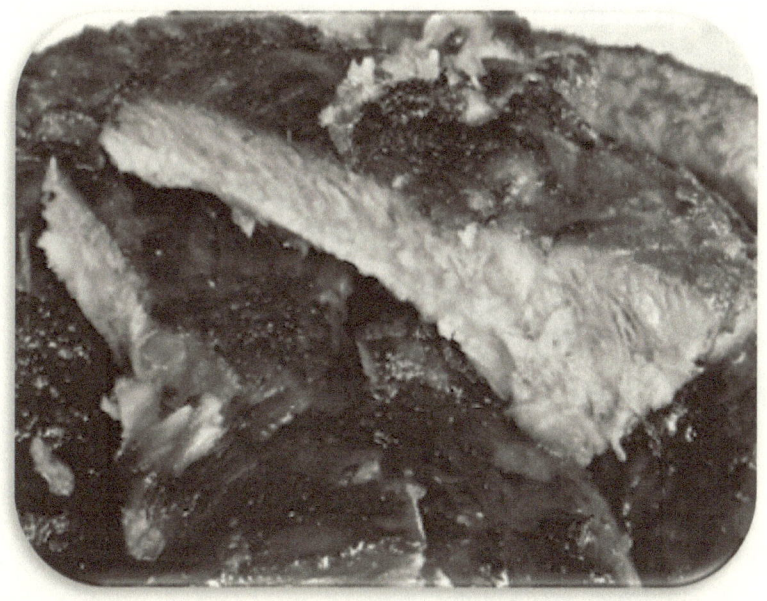

Egg Fried Rice

Prep Time: 15minutes

Cook Time: 10 minutes

Serves: 6

Ingredients

3 tablespoons of oil

1/4 cup chopped green onion

2 cloves garlic, minced

1/2 cup cooked pork, chopped

4 cups cooked rice

1 teaspoon low-salt soy sauce

1/2 cup frozen green peas

6 eggs, scrambled &chopped

1/4 teaspoon dry mustard

Directions:

1. In a large skillet, heat oil over medium heat. Add the garlic and cook until tender.

2. Add the onion, stir and cook 2 minutes.

3. Add the pork, the rice as well as soy sauce. Stir thoroughly and cook 3 minutes.

4. Add the rest of the ingredients; cook until thoroughly heated.

Nutritional Facts Per Serving: 1 Cup Per Serving

Calories: 270 kcals

Potassium: 202 mg

Phosphorus: 173mg

Sodium: 118mg

Protein: 12 g

Calcium: 3mg

Carbohydrates: 38g

Fat: 8g

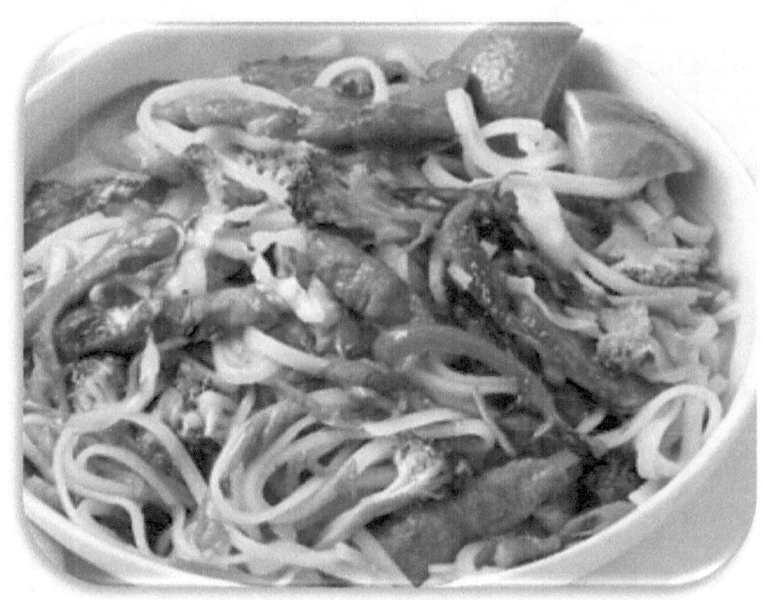

Pork Stir-Fry With Noodles

Pork Stir-Fry With Noodles

Prep Time: minutes

Cook Time: minutes

Serves: 2

Ingredients

8 oz. lean pork fillet, thinly cut

2 medium carrots, pre-boiled &drained

1 small red pepper, pre-boiled &drained

1 medium zucchini, pre-boiled & drained

½ teaspoon of Thai seven spice powder

Olive oil, for frying

Directions

1. Place pork fillets in a little oil and fry in a pan.

2. Cut the vegetables into strips and add to the pan.

3. Add the Thai Spice powder and stir-fry until the pork the well- cooked.

4. Serve with noodles.

Nutritional Facts Per Serving:

Calories: 280kcals

Potassium: 24mg

Phosphorus: 13mg

Sodium: 6mg

Protein: 39g

Fat: 11g

Cranberry Pork Roast

Prep Time: 10 minutes

Cook Time: 10 hrs.

Serves: 12

Ingredients

4 lb center cut pork roast

1 cup cranberries, chopped

1 teaspoon black pepper

1 tablespoon brown sugar

¼ cup honey

1 teaspoon grated orange peel

⅛ teaspoon of nutmeg

⅛ teaspoon of ground cloves

Directions

1. Sprinkle the pork roast with pepper and place in a slow cooker.

2. Add together the rest of the ingredients and pour over the roast.

3. Cover pot and cook for 10 hours on low.

4. Remove, slice into 24 pieces and top with drippings from pot.

Nutritional Facts Per Serving: Serving size: 2/3 cup

Calories: 192 kcals

Potassium: 359mg

Phosphorus: 214mg

Sodium: 122mg

Calcium: 21mg

Protein: 21g

Carbohydrates: 13 g

Fat: 9 g

Cholesterol: 70 mg

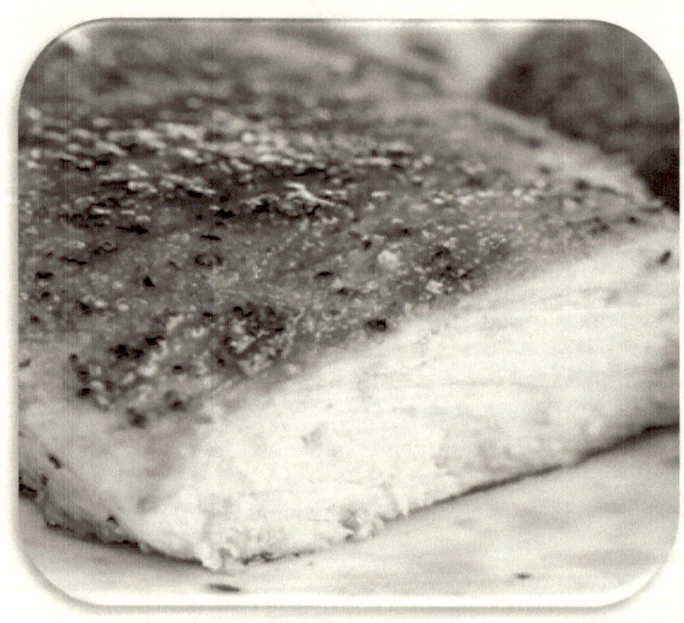

Pork chops

Pork Chops

Prep Time: 15minutes

Cook Time: 40minutes

Serves: 6

Ingredients

6 pork loin (3 oz. each)

2 tablespoons of flour

2 teaspoon of margarine

½ teaspoon of basil

½ teaspoon of rosemary

½ teaspoon of sage

1 ½ cup onions, sliced

1/8 teaspoon of pepper

1 cup water

Directions

1. Coat flour chops with flour.

2. Melt the margarine in a large skillet and brown the coated chops over medium-high heat.

3. Add onions, basil, rosemary, sage, pepper and water.

5. Cover and let it simmer for 30 minutes.

Pork Chops With Herb Crust

Prep Time: 20minutes

Cook Time: 25minutes

Serves: 2

Ingredients

2 pork chops, trimmed of fat

2 teaspoon oil

1 teaspoon mustard

2 spring onions, chopped finely

1 clove garlic, crushed

2 tablespoons breadcrumbs

1 pinch chopped parsley

Directions

1. Preheat the oven to 400°F.

2. Spread the mustard over each of the pork chop (one side only) and place in a baking dish or

3. Combine the parsley, breadcrumbs, oil, garlic and onions together and press the mixture over each pork chop and cover with foil.

4. Place in the oven and bake for 25 minutes. Serve with boiled potatoes.

Pork With Pear Chutney

Prep Time: 10minutes

Cook Time: 35minutes

Serves: 4

Ingredients

1 red onion, chopped

2 pears, cores off & chopped

1/3 cup red wine vinegar

1/3 cup brown sugar, firmly packed

1 tablespoon olive oil

½ teaspoon dried chili flakes

4 medium pork chops

Serving:

4 small corn cobs, boiled

2 cups of boiled green beans, chopped

12 asparagus spears, boiled

Directions

1. Bring pear, vinegar, onion, sugar and chili to a boil in a saucepan.

2. Simmer on low heat for 20 minutes until the pear is soft, stirring occasionally.

3. In the meantime, brown pork chops in oil for 4 minutes on each side.

4. To serve, divide the green beans, corn, and asparagus between 4 plates and place the brown pork chops on them. Top with the pear chutney.

Nutritional Facts Per Serving: Pork chop with all servings (pear chutney, beans, corn, & asparagus)

Calories: 310.7kcals

Potassium: 1075mg

Phosphorus: 440mg

Sodium: 125mg

Protein: 35g

Carbohydrates: 50g

Fat: 12g

Beef Main Dishes

Beef & Mushroom Casserole

Prep Time: 20 minutes

Cook Time: 2 hrs.

Serves: 6

Ingredients

1 tablespoon olive oil

35 oz. lean topside steak, cubed (2 inches)

¼ teaspoon dried thyme leaves

Ground pepper

Sprinkle of ground cloves

1 medium onion, sliced

2 bay leaves

4 medium carrots, peeled & chopped

1 cup parsnip, chopped & peeled

1 ½ cups dry red wine

2 cups beef stock

22/3 cup of button mushrooms, halved

2 teaspoons cornflour

½ teaspoon grated nutmeg

2 tablespoons brandy

Directions

1. Heat the oil in a large saucepan over medium heat.

2. Add the beef cubes in batches until well browned.

3. Add in the thyme, pepper, ground, onion, cloves and bay leaves. Stir and cook for about 5 minutes or until the onion is soft.

3. Add the parsnip carrots, stock and wine and bring to a boil. Cover, set heat to low and simmer with occasional stir, for 1 hour 30 minutes. If it becomes too dry, add more water.

4 Raise the lid and add in the mushrooms. Cook again for 10 minutes.

5. Now add the cornflour mixed with 2 teaspoons of water to thicken the sauce.

6. Add the nutmeg and brandy and more pepper, if needed.

7. Heat it through and then remove.

8. Enjoy the casserole with rice and beans, if desired.

Nutritional Facts Per Serving:

Calories: 310kcals

Potassium: 980mg

Phosphorus: 420mg

Sodium: 360mg

Protein: 40g

Carbohydrates: 7g

Fat: 9g

Onion- Packed Steak

Prep Time: 15 minutes

Cook Time: 1 hr. 15 minutes

Serves: 8

Ingredients

1/4 cup flour

1/8 teaspoon pepper

2 tablespoons oil

1 1/2 lb. round steak, ¾" thick

1 cup water

1 clove garlic, minced

1 tablespoon vinegar

1 bay leaf

3 medium onions, sliced

1/4 teaspoon dried thyme, crushed

Directions:

1. First, cut the steak into 8 equal sizes.

2. Next, mix the flour and pepper together and then pound into meat.

3. In a skillet, brown meat in oil on both sides. Remove and set aside.

4. Add water to the skillet as well as the vinegar, thyme and bay leaf. Let it boil and then add in the reserve meat.

5. Add the sliced onions, cover and let it simmer for an hour.

Nutritional Facts Per Serving: 2 oz Meat Per Serving

Calories: 271kcals

Potassium: 369mg

Phosphorus: 180mg

Sodium: 45mg

Protein: 18g

Carbohydrates: 7g

Fat: 19g

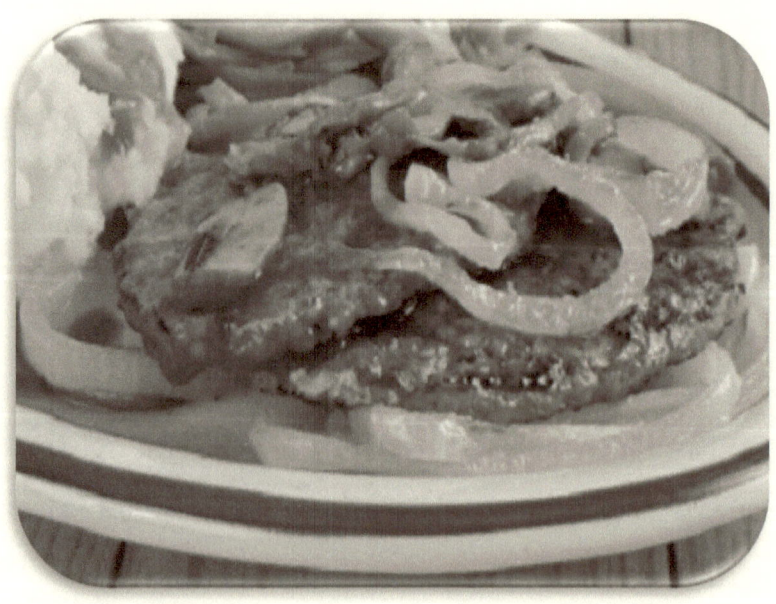

Texas Hash

Prep Time: 10 minutes

Cook Time: 60 minutes

Serves: 4

Ingredients

16 oz. minced beef

1 large onion, chopped

1 tin tomatoes

2 tablespoons of rice

1 green pepper, deseeded & sliced thinly

1 tablespoon Worcestershire sauce

1 teaspoon of sugar

Pepper

Olive oil

Directions

1. Add a small quantity of olive oil to a pan; set heat to medium and sauté the onion until golden.

2. Add the mince, stir to break up and then add the pepper, stirring thoroughly to mix.

3. Empty the entire content of tomatoes to the pan; add the Worcestershire sauce as well as the rice. Stir and cook a couple of minutes until the liquid reduces slightly.

4. Transfer to a greased dish and cook on medium heat for 45 minutes at a temperature of 356°F.

Spicy Beef Stir-Fry

Prep Time: 10 minutes

Cook Time: 60 minutes

Serves: 4

<u>Ingredients</u>

¼ teaspoon sesame oil

2 tablespoons cornstarch

2 tablespoons water

½ teaspoon sugar

1 large egg, beaten

3 tablespoons canola oil

1 cup green bell peppers, sliced

12 oz. beef round tip, sliced

1 cup onions, sliced

Ground red chili pepper, to taste

1 tablespoon sherry

2 teaspoons reduced sodium soy sauce

<u>Directions</u>

1. Combine a tablespoon of cornstarch and a tablespoon of water together in a bowl. Whisk in the beaten egg, beef and a tablespoon of canola oil and let it marinate for 15-20 minutes.

2. Combine the rest of the cornstarch and water in a separate bowl and set aside.

3. Heat the 2 tablespoons of canola oil that's left in a large skillet and add in the meat mixture. Let it cook until the meat starts to brown and then add the bell peppers, chili pepper and onion.

4. Add sherry, sauté a minute and then add the sugar, sesame oil and soy sauce. Add the cornstarch mix to thicken it.

5. Serve, garnished with parsley, if desired.

Nutritional Facts Per Serving:

Calories: 285kcals

Potassium: 429mg

Phosphorus: 215mg

Sodium: 176mg

Calcium: 38mg

Protein: 20g

Carbohydrates:10 g

Fat: 18g

Cholesterol: 99mg

Beef And Barley Stew

Prep Time: 1 hr. 30 minutes

Cook Time: 2 hrs. 30 minutes

Serves: 6

Ingredients

1 cup of uncooked pearl barley

1 lb. lean beef stew meat, cut into cubes of 1 ½"

2 tablespoons of flour

½ teaspoon salt

¼ teaspoon black pepper

2 tbsp. oil

½ cup onion, diced

1 clove garlic, minced

1 large stalk celery, sliced

2 carrots, sliced ¼" thick

1 teaspoon herb seasoning, preferably Mrs. Dash

2 bay leaves

Directions

1. Begin by soaking the barley in 2 cups of water for at least 1 hour.

2. In a plastic bag, place the flour and the black pepper as well as the stew meat. Shake bag to coat the stew meat with the flour.

3. In a large pot, brown the stew meat in oil and then remove.

4. Now add the onion, garlic and the celery and sauté in the meat drippings for 2 minutes.

5. Pour in 8 cups of water, bring to a boil and then return meat to the pan. Add the salt and bay leaves. Lower heat.

6. Once simmering, drain the barley and rinse. Add it to the pot. Cover and cook an hour, but every 15 minutes, open pot and stir.

7. After 1 hour, add the carrots and seasoning. Simmer 1 hour.

Savory Mince

Prep Time: 10 minutes

Cook Time: 30minutes

Serves: 4

Ingredients

18 oz. lean beef or lamb, minced

1 tablespoon of sunflower oil

1 small (2½ oz.) onion, chopped finely

1 large clove garlic

1oz of flour

11/4 cup of water

1 teaspoon of ground black pepper

½ tin (8oz) chopped tomatoes

2 teaspoons of dried basil

Directions

1. Add oil to a large saucepan on medium heat. Add the onion and fry until translucent.

2. Add the mince, stir and fry and then drain the fat.

3. Remove from heat. Add flour to the pan, drained tomatoes, half of the water and the herbs.

4. Place lid on and let it simmer 1 hour until tender. Gradually add the remaining water as the mince thickens.

5. Cool and serve.

Nutritional Facts Per Serving: Calories: 315kcals

Potassium: 312mg; Phosphorus: 8.5 mg; Sodium: 0.3mg

Protein: 21g; Carbohydrates: 8g Fat: 21g

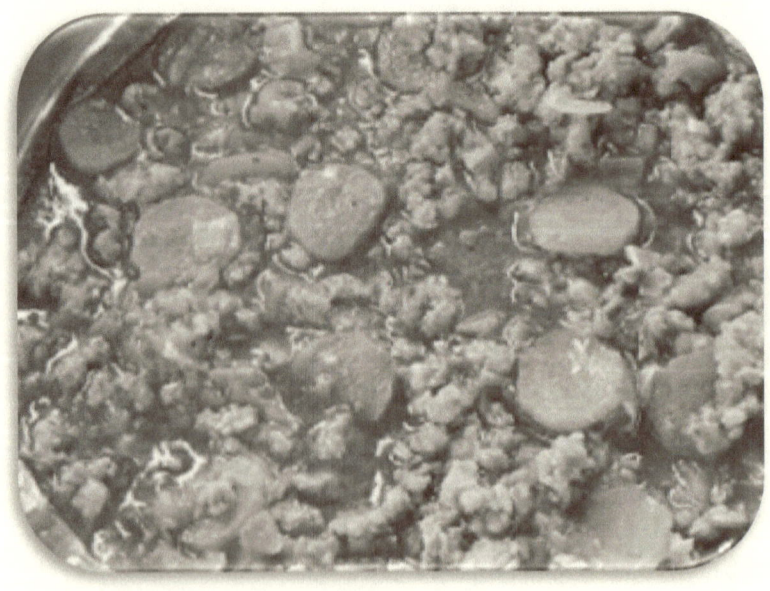

BBQ Baby Back Ribs

Prep Time: 15minutes

Cook Time: 2 hrs.

Serves: 12

Ingredients

2 slabs (about 3½ lb.) baby back ribs

12 mini-ears corn on the cob

1 portion of rub

1 teaspoon black pepper

1 cup packed dark brown sugar

1 teaspoon red pepper flakes

2 teaspoons garlic powder

1 teaspoon smoked paprika

2 teaspoons dark chili powder

2 teaspoons dehydrated onion flakes

Directions

1. Preheat your oven to 400°F.

2. Combine all the spice ingredients in a bowl and rub mixture on both sides of the meat.

3. Place ribs on wire rack tray and wrap with tightly with foil. Bake for 11/2 to 2 hours, remove, take off foil and use tongs to set aside ribs.

4. Drain the liquid from the pan off and return the rib to the tray. Cook 15 until crispy.

5. Let it sit 10 minutes. Cut and serve. (Place the corn on the cob in a dish, pour in half inch water, cover with plastic wrap and microwave on high for 5 minutes). Enjoy!

Nutritional Facts Per Serving: Calories: 324kcals

Potassium: 453mg; Phosphorus: 198 mg; Sodium: 102mg

Calcium: 47mg; Protein: 18g; Carbohydrates: 33g

Fat: 15g; Cholesterol: 58mg

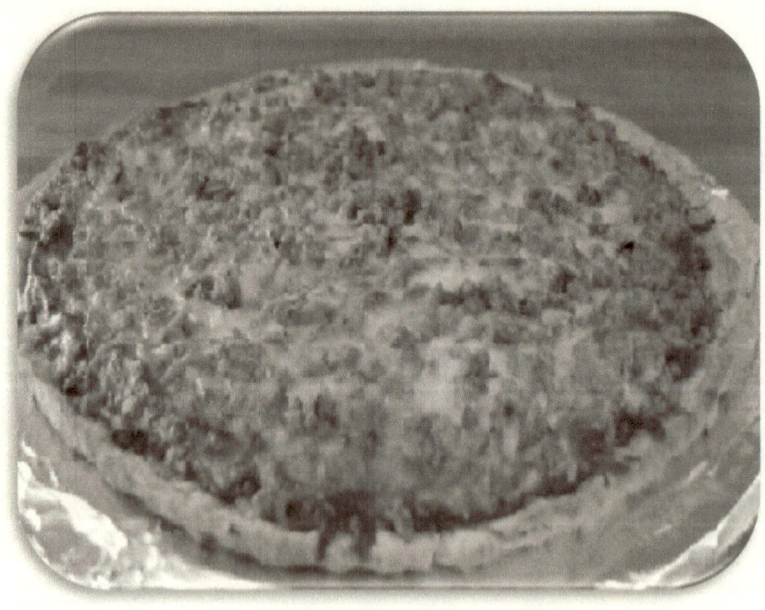

Low sodium pizza

Low Sodium Pizza

Prep Time: 15minutes

Cook Time: 40 minutes

Serves: 12

Ingredients

2 cups of all-purpose flour

1 cup warm water

1 teaspoon instant yeast

1 tablespoon sugar

6 oz. mozzarella cheese, shredded

1 tablespoon canola oil

½ lb. ground beef, cooked & well- drained

¼ cup green pepper, chopped

¼ cup onion, chopped

1 tablespoon canola oil

½ teaspoon oregano

1/3 teaspoon garlic powder

½ cup water

75 ml unsalted tomato sauce

Directions

1. Preheat oven to 400°F.

2. Add yeast to warm water to dissolve. Add the oil and sugar. Gradually add in the flour and stir to make a soft dough.

3. Place the dough in a greased bowl and cover it. Let it rest for 15-20 minutes.

4. In a small saucepan, add together the garlic powder, tomato sauce, oregano, oil and water. Simmer on low heat for 5 minutes.

3. Press dough on a greased baking sheet and over the edges. Pour the sauce over it and then top with green pepper, onion, beef and cheese.

4. Bake in the oven for 30 minutes until golden brown. Cut into pieces and serve.

Nutritional Facts Per Serving:

Calories: 201 kcals

Potassium: 176mg

Phosphorus: 115mg

Sodium: 75mg

Protein: 11 g

Carbohydrates: 19g

Beef Casserole

Prep Time: 15minutes

Cook Time: 60 minutes

Serves: 4

Ingredients

18oz lean beef

1 medium onion (6 oz.), chopped

2 medium carrots, peeled & sliced

11/4 cup water

1 tablespoon of vegetable oil

¼ teaspoon white pepper

¼ teaspoon salt

1 tablespoon fresh parsley, chopped

Directions

1. Add oil to the pan and sauté the onion until brown.

2. Add the beef, fry and then add water. Simmer until beef is almost cooked.

Add the carrots and keep simmering until well-cooked.

3. Add salt and pepper to taste. Garnish with chopped parsley and serve with boiled rice.

Nutritional Facts Per Serving: Calories: 304kcals

Potassium: 456mg; Phosphorus: 202 mg; Sodium: 102mg

Protein: 23g; Carbohydrates: 33g; Fat: 15g Salt: 0.5g

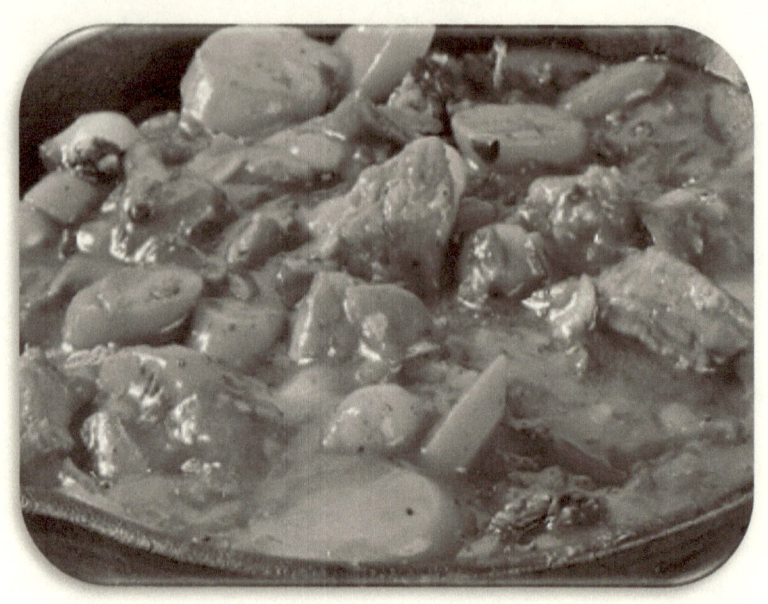

Chili Rice With Beef

Prep Time: 15minutes

Cook Time: 15minutes

Serves: 4

Ingredients

1 pound lean ground beef

2 tablespoons vegetable oil

1 cup onion, chopped

1 ½ teaspoons chili seasoning powder

2 cups rice, cooked

¼ cup chopped celery

⅛ teaspoon black pepper

½ teaspoon sage

Directions

1. Heat the oil in the pan; add the beef and onion and cook with occasional stirring, until browned.

2. Add the rest of the ingredients and combine well.

3. Remove from heat. Cover and set aside for about 10 minutes.

Nutritional Facts Per Serving: Serving size: 1 cup

Calories: 360 kcals

Potassium: 427mg

Phosphorus: 233mg

Sodium: 78mg

Calcium: 34mg

Protein: 23g

Carbohydrates: 26g

Fat: 26g

Cholesterol: 65 mg

Peppercorn Steak

Prep Time: minutes

Cook Time: minutes

Serves: 2

Ingredients

4oz beef steaks

4oz half fat crème fraiche

Freshly ground black pepper

2 teaspoons vegetable oil

2 teaspoons peppercorns, crushed

Directions

1. Add the oil to a large non-stick pan and heat.

2. Season the steaks with the black pepper and cook for about 5 minutes over medium heat.

3. Remove the steaks and place on warm platters.

4. Add the peppercorns and crème fraîche to the pan. Cook and stir for 2 minutes or until thickened.

5. Spoon 1 or 2 tablespoons of sauce over the steak and serve with preferred boiled vegetables.

Seafood Main Dishes

Salmon Mornay

Prep Time: 15 minutes

Cook Time: 50minutes

Serves: 6

Ingredients

3 cups of boiled white rice

1 large onion, diced

21 oz. canned pink salmon, drained & chopped

¾ cup corn kernels

2 tablespoons margarine, salt reduced

3 tablespoons of plain flour

2 cups reduced fat milk

2 tablespoons of fresh breadcrumbs

Pepper, to taste

½ cup of grated parmesan cheese

2 tablespoons fresh parsley, roughly chopped

For the Salad:

6 rings green capsicum

6 lettuce leaves

24 slices of cucumber

1 large stick celery

6 teaspoons of Italian dressing, fat free

Directions:

1. Place the cooked rice in a lightly greased nonstick baking dish and set aside.

2. In a large saucepan, melt the margarine and add the onion, stirring until soft.

3. Add the flour, stir to mix and then add in the milk. Stir until bubbling and then lower heat and keep stirring until the sauce thickens.

3. Add the pink salmon as well as the corn and pepper. Stir to combine well and if too thick, add a little milk.

4. Now pour the salmon mixture over the rice in the baking dish and top it with breadcrumbs, parsley and grated cheese.

5. Bake for 30 minutes. Remove once golden brown and serve, if desired with green salad.

Nutritional Facts Per Serving: 1 chicken thigh

Calories: 449kcals

Potassium: 580mg

Phosphorus: 489mg

Sodium: 520mg

Protein: 33g

Carbohydrates: 40g

Fat: 17g

Tuna & Lemon Pasta

Prep Time: 10minutes

Cook Time: 30minutes

Serves: 4

Ingredients

17.5 ounce bow pasta (farfalle)

1 tablespoon olive oil

1 Spanish onion, diced

15 oz. tinned tuna, drained &flaked

½ cup parmesan cheese, freshly grated

2 cups boiled broccoli florets

Rind and juice of 2 lemons

½ cup light sour cream

Black pepper

1 tablespoon capers (optional)

1 tablespoon shaved parmesan, extra

Directions:

1. In a large saucepan, bring lots of water to a boil, add the pasta and cook until tender. Drain pan and set aside.

2. In the same saucepan, heat oil and add in onion, tuna, broccoli, parmesan, lemon juice and rind as well as black pepper.

3. Return the drained pasta to the tuna mixture. Add the sour cream, stir and heat through.

4. Serve with a sprinkling of capers and shaved Parmesan.

Nutritional Facts Per Serving: serving size- 1/6 chicken &1/2 cup rice

Calories: 444.5 kcals

Potassium: 550mg

Phosphorus: 430mg

Sodium: 425mg

Protein: 38g

Carbohydrates: 27g

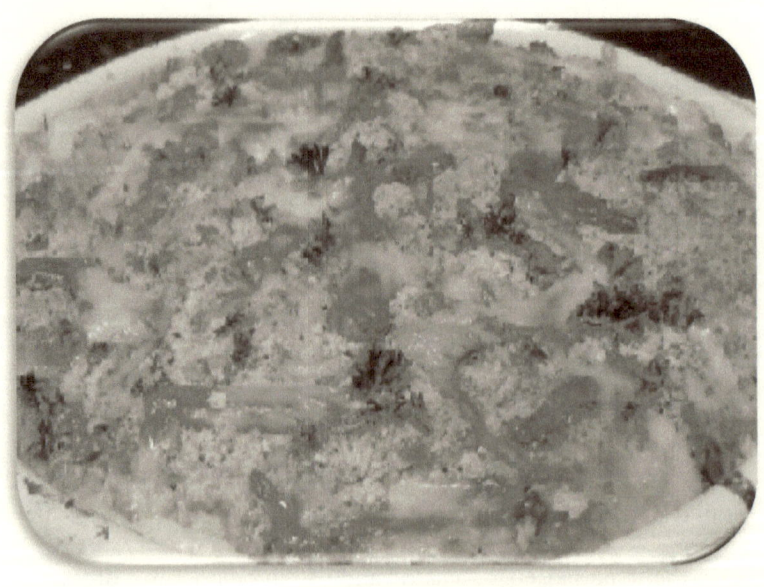

Salmon Mornay

Cod Fillet With Lemon Sauce

Prep Time: 15minutes

Cook Time: 15minutes

Serves: 4

Ingredients

4 medium (4 oz.) cod fillets

1 lemon, grated rind and Juice

1 heaped tablespoon of corn flour

1 tablespoon unsalted butter

4 tablespoons of water

¼ teaspoon black pepper

Directions

1. Add the water, lemon rind and juice to a small saucepan and bring to the boil.

2. Combine corn flour with water, add to the saucepan to thicken. Season with salt and pepper.

3. Grill the fish with butter for 5 minutes.

4. Serve with the sauce as a side, or simply pour the sauce over the fish and enjoy!

Nutritional Facts Per Serving: Calories: 151 kcals

Potassium: 406mg; Phosphorus: 207mg; Sodium: 300mg

Protein: 21g; Carbohydrates: 7g

Spicy Pesto Catfish

Prep Time: 30minutes

Cook Time: 25minutes

Serves: 6

Ingredients

2 pounds catfish (boned &cut into fillets) 6 5-oz. pieces

4 teaspoons pesto

½ cup mozzarella cheese

¾ cup panko bread crumbs

2 tablespoons olive oil

1 teaspoon onion powder

1 teaspoon garlic powder

½ teaspoon dried oregano

½ teaspoon black pepper

½ teaspoon red pepper flakes

Directions:

1. Preheat your oven to 400°F.

2. Combine all the seasoning ingredients in a bowl and sprinkle evenly on fish on both sides.

3. Spread a teaspoon of pesto on the filets and set aside.

4. Combine the breadcrumbs, oil and cheese in a bowl. Coat the fish in the mixture (pesto side only).

5. Grease baking tray with a generous amount of oil. Place in the fish, with the pesto side up and bake 20 minutes until browned.

6. Set aside for 10 minutes.

Nutritional Facts Per Serving:

Calories: 238kcals

Potassium: 385mg

Phosphorus: 285 mg

Sodium: 255mg

Calcium: 89mg

Protein: 21g

Carbohydrates: 8g

Fat: 15g

Cholesterol: 58mg

SNACKS & DESSERTS

Snacks play a vital role in a healthy kidney diet. Whether on dialysis or in the early stages, snacking should regularly feature in your diet. It is helpful for curbing appetite and preventing overeating at subsequent meals. Snacking should be low in sodium and involve kidney- friendly fruits such as apples, blue berries, strawberries, carrot sticks, grapes and raspberries.

For those with sweet tooth, desserts can be made renal- friendly, with just the right nutrients that will be helpful for your kidney. You can enjoy your cakes and cookies with ease.

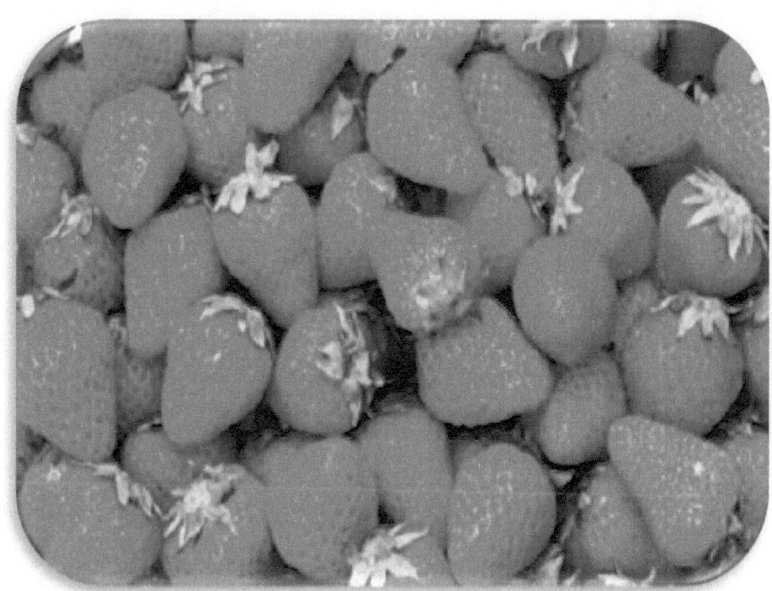

Snacks

Spicy Apple Juice

Prep Time: 5minutes

Cook Time: 20minutes

Serves: 8

Ingredients

12 whole cloves

½ teaspoon nutmeg

4 cinnamon sticks, broken

1 quart apple, unsweetened

¼ teaspoon allspice

Directions

1. Combine all the ingredients in saucepan.

2. Bring to boil on medium heat simmer 20 minutes.

3. Pass through a strainer and serve in cups.

Nutritional Facts Per Serving: Serving size: ½ cup

Calories: 63

Potassium: 132 mg; Phosphorus: 10 mg

Sodium: 6 mg; Protein: 1g; Calcium: 18 mg

Carbohydrates: 15g; Fat: 1g

Fresh Fruit Compote

Prep Time: 10 minutes

Cook Time: 0minutes

Serves: 8

Ingredients

1/2 cup blackberries

1/2 cup strawberries

1/2 cup blueberries

1/2 cup peaches, pared & cut

1/4 cup red raspberries, sweetened, not thawed

1/2 cup orange juice, unsweetened

1 apple, cut into pieces

1 banana, cut into pieces

Directions

1. Pour the orange juice into a large container and add the rest of the ingredients.

Nutritional Facts Per Serving: ½ cup per serving

Calories: 44kcals

Potassium: 140mg; Phosphorus: 13 mg; Sodium: 1mg

Protein: .5g; Carbohydrates: 11g; Fat: .2g

Garlic Oyster Crackers

Prep Time: minutes

Cook Time: minutes

Serves: 14

Ingredients

½ c. popcorn oil, butter-flavored

1 tablespoons of garlic powder

2 teaspoons of dried dill weed

7 c. oyster crackers

Directions

1. Preheat your oven to 250°F.

2. Combine the oil and the garlic powder in a bowl. Add the crackers, stir to coat evenly.

3. Sprinkle dill weed over and toss to mix.

4. Spread crackers on baking tray and bake 45 minutes, gently mixing every 15 minutes.

5 cool on paper towels and store in an airtight container.

Nutritional Facts Per Serving: Serving size: ½ cup

Calories: 118kcals

Potassium: 21mg

Phosphorus: 15 mg

Sodium: 166mg

Protein: 2g

Carbohydrates: 12g

Fat: 7g

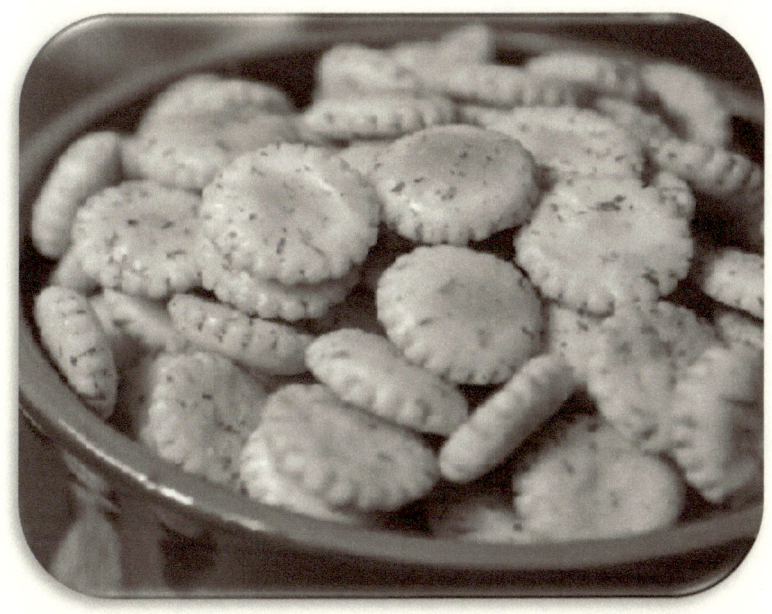

Desserts

Baked Custard

Prep Time: 10 minutes

Cook Time: 30 minutes

Serves: 1

Ingredients

1/2 cup low-fat milk (2%)

1 egg

1/8 teaspoon vanilla

1/8 teaspoon nutmeg

Artificial sweetener, to taste

Directions:

1. Scald milk, cool slightly and then break egg into small bowl.

2. Beat in nutmeg, add the scalded milk as well as vanilla and sweetener and combine thoroughly.

3. Set bowl in a baking pan. Add water to the pan and bake for 30 minutes at a temperature of 325°F.

Nutritional Facts Per Serving:

Calories: 135kcals

Potassium: 249mg

Phosphorus: 205 mg

Sodium: 124mg

Protein: 10g

Carbohydrates: 7g

Fat: 7g

Cholesterol: 58mg

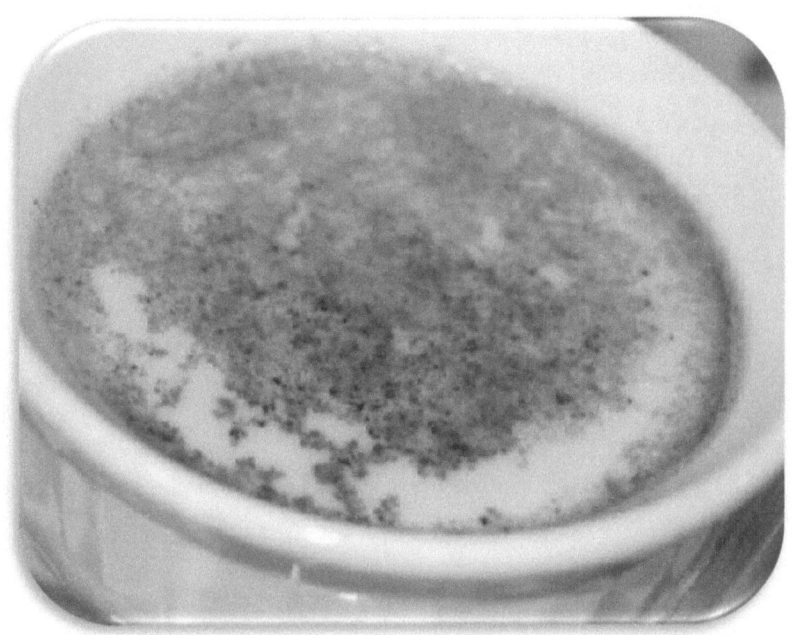

Chinese Almond Cookies

Prep Time: 10 minutes

Cook Time: 10 minutes

Serves: 24

Ingredients

1 cup margarine, softened

1 egg

1 cup sugar

3 cups flour

1 teaspoon baking soda

1 teaspoon almond extract

Directions:

1. Cream the sugar and margarine and then beat in the egg and mix thoroughly.

2. Dry the sifted dry ingredients as well as the almond extract and mix to combine well.

3. Make balls of about ¾ inches diameter and press a hole in the center of each of them.

4. Place in the oven and bake for 10 minutes at 400°F until golden brown.

Nutritional Facts Per Serving: 3 Cookies Per Serving

Calories: 158kcals

Potassium: 18mg

Phosphorus: 17mg

Sodium: 99mg

Protein: 2g

Carbohydrates: 20g

Fat: 8g

Low Sodium Pound Cake

Prep Time: 10minutes

Cook Time: 30minutes

Serves:

Ingredients

3/4 cup sugar

1/4 lb. butter, unsalted

2 large eggs, slightly beaten

1 1/4 cup bread flour

3 ounce milk

Directions

1. Cream butter and add sugar gradually. Beat until fluffy.

2. Add the eggs, milk and flour and then mix thoroughly.

3. Place in a lined baking pan and bake for 30 minutes at 375 F.

Nutritional Facts Per Serving: 1/9 cup per serving

Calories: 243kcals

Potassium: 47mg

Phosphorus: 45 mg

Sodium: 18mg

Protein: 3.7g

Carbohydrates: 31g

Fat: 12g

Cholesterol: 75 mg

Cinnamon Crisps
Prep Time: 5 minutes

Cook Time: 7 minutes

Serves: 4

Ingredients

1/2 teaspoon vanilla

1 tablespoon hot water

1 1/2 tablespoons sugar

4 6-inch flour tortillas

1 teaspoon cinnamon

2 tablespoons margarine, melted

Directions:

1. Add together the vanilla and water in a bowl and stir well to mix. Add the cinnamon and sugar and stir thoroughly.

2. Brush tortillas with margarine on both sides and brush each side with the water mixture.

3. Sprinkle tortillas with the sugar mixture and place on a wire rack in a jelly roll pan.

4. Bake for 7 minutes at 400F

Nutritional Facts Per Serving: 3 Cookies Per Serving

Calories: 168kcals

Potassium: 35mg, Sodium: 83mg

Protein: 3g, Carbohydrates: 21g

Fat: 8g

Chocolate Strawberries

Prep Time: minutes

Cook Time: minutes

Serves: 18

Ingredients

1/2 cup semi-sweet chocolate chips

1 tablespoon corn syrup

5 tablespoon margarine

1 qt Strawberries, washed & dried.

Directions

1. Place the chocolate chips, corn syrup and margarine in a pan and melt over low heat. Stir to smoothen.

2. Remove and place in a pan of water.

3. Dip the strawberries into the chocolate mix; place on waxed paper and chill.

Nutritional Facts Per Serving: Serving size: 2 each

Calories: 69kcals

Potassium: 70mg

Phosphorus: 14mg

Sodium: 40mg

Protein: .5g

Carbohydrates: 6.6g

Fat: 5g

Cholesterol: 0 mg

Vanilla Ice Cream

Prep Time: 15minutes

Cook Time: 3 hr.

Serves: 6

Ingredients

3 (2 oz.) egg yolks

4 oz. caster sugar

1 cup milk

1 teaspoon vanilla essence

½ cup double cream

Directions

1. Add the egg yolks and sugar to a mixing bowl, and beat until creamy.

2. Heat up the milk, add in the vanilla essence and add to the eggs mix, stirring thoroughly.

3. Strain into a bowl over a pan of hot and simmering water and cook for 30 minutes on moderate heat. Stir constantly until thickened but do not boil mixture.

4. Cool and then add in the cream, stirring well.

5. Pour into an ice tray.

Nutritional Facts Per Serving: Serving size: 2 each

Calories: 257kcals

Potassium: 105mg

Phosphorus: 105mg

Sodium: .8mg

Protein: 3.5g

Carbohydrates: 21g

Fat: 18g

Cholesterol: 0 mg

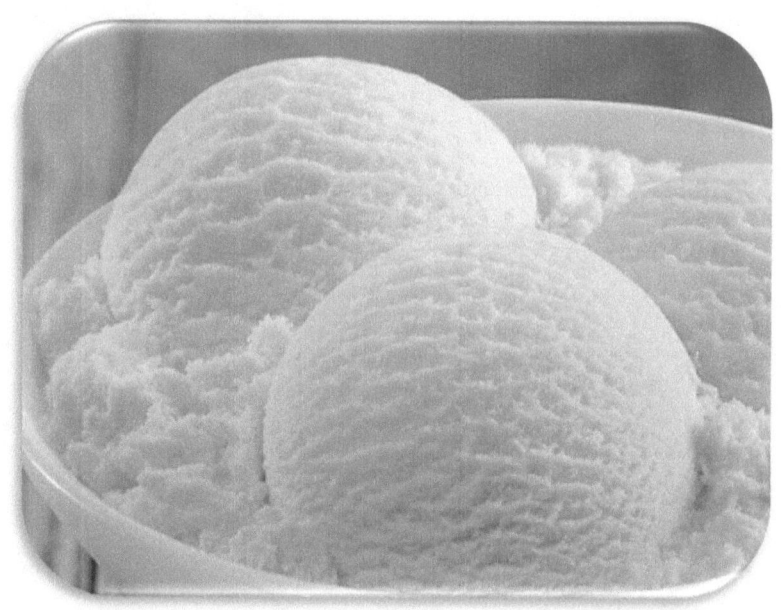

Maple Crisp Bars

Prep Time: minutes

Cook Time: 0 minutes

Serves: 20

Ingredients

1 cup sugar

1/3 cup margarine

1/2 cup of maple pancake syrup

1 teaspoon of maple extract

8 cups puffed rice cereal

Directions:

1. Melt margarine in a large saucepan over medium heat. Add sugar, syrup and extract. Stir and bring to a boil and then remove from heat.

2. Add the cereal and stir so that it coats with sugar mixture.

3. Place into a greased baking pan and refrigerate. Cut into 20 bars.

Nutritional Facts Per Serving:

Calories: 110kcals

Potassium: 10mg

Phosphorus: 6 mg

Sodium: 83mg

Protein: 0g

Carbohydrates: 21g

Fat: 3g

Cinnamon Rice Pudding

Prep Time: 5minutes

Cook Time: 60 minutes

Serves: 4

Ingredients

4 oz. pudding rice

11/4 cup whole milk

1 cup double cream

11/4 cup water

3 oz. sugar

1 teaspoon vanilla extract

1 teaspoon ground cinnamon

Directions:

1. Combine all the ingredients in a pan; but set aside the cinnamon and vanilla essence.

2. Let it heat for 1 hour on low heat and stir frequently to prevent rice from sticking to the bottom.

3. Once rice is done, add the vanilla essence and season with cinnamon, stirring and heating for an extra 10 minutes.

Nutritional Facts Per Serving:

Calories: 586kcals

Potassium: 192mg

Phosphorus: 136 mg

Sodium: .1mg

Protein: 5g

Carbohydrates: 46g

Fat: 43g

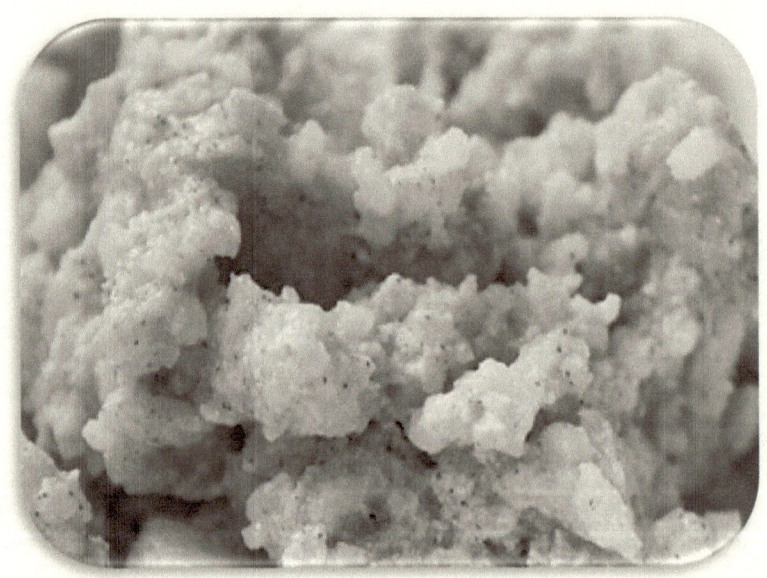

Strawberry Ice Cream

Prep Time: minutes

Cook Time: minutes

Serves: 6

Ingredients

1 10-oz package sweetened strawberries, frozen

1 cup crushed ice

1 tablespoon lemon juice

3/4 cup non-dairy coffee creamer

1/2 cup sugar

1-2 drops of red food coloring

Directions:

1. Thaw strawberries.

2. Blend ingredients in a blender until smooth.

3. Pour into a dish, cover and place in the freezer to solidify.

Nutritional Facts Per Serving:

Calories: 144kcals

Potassium: 108mg

Phosphorus: 25 mg

Sodium: 25mg

Protein: 1g

Carbohydrates: 28g

Fat: 3g

The End

www.ingramcontent.com/pod-product-compliance
Lightning Source LLC
Chambersburg PA
CBHW021816170526
45157CB00007B/2609